Chemical Pharmacy Enters the University

Chemical Pharmacy Enters the University

Johannes Hartmann and the Didactic Care of *Chymiatria* in the Early Seventeenth Century

by Bruce T. Moran

American Institute of the History of Pharmacy
Madison, Wisconsin
1991

I.S.B.N. 0-931292-23-9 pbk.
I.S.B.N. 0-931292-24-7

Publication No. 14 (New Series)
Gregory J. Higby and Elaine C. Stroud, General Editors

COVER: Johannes Hartmann (1568–1631) from Wilhelm Dilich, *Urbs et Academia Marpurgensis . . . Professorum Marpurgensium Icones* . . . edidit Ferdinandus Justi (1898)

An Urdang Publication
on International Trends in Pharmaceutical History

second in a series dedicated to the memory of
GEORGE URDANG
(1882–1960)

Historian of Pharmacy and Founding Director (1941–1957)
of the American Institute of the History of Pharmacy

In Memory of My Father

Contents

Introduction

The subject of this book is the emergence of an academic discipline called *chymiatria* (chemical medicine) in the early seventeenth century. The coming into being of that discipline at the German University of Marburg is an important event in the history of pharmacy. Instruction in the preparation of medicines, many of the chemical sort, gained a formal place within the university curriculum for the first time. As an independent subject laying claim to its own intellectual and physical spaces within the university, chemical pharmacy acquired the status at Marburg of an institutionalized study. The first appointed professor of *chymiatria* was Johannes Hartmann (1568–1631) and, as we shall see, it was due to Hartmann that the new discipline received its ideological identity.

In the study that follows, we will focus first on the conditions that brought *chymiatria* into the university. We can explore the discipline's philosophical underpinnings best by examining a controversy that arose between Hartmann and one of the most well-known practical chemists of the day, Andreas Libavius (1540–1616). Thereafter, our attention will shift to the practical content of *chymiatria*. Very little is known about what instructors actually taught in courses dealing with the preparation of chemical medicines in the early seventeenth century. For that reason, a laboratory diary kept over two terms at Marburg survives as an informative and historiographically valuable document. It serves as a guide into Hartmann's laboratory and offers a means to describe the actual scope and content of the Marburg course in chemical medicine.

Exploring the philosophical and pedagogical sides of *chymiatria* raises the important question of how Paracelsian philosophy relates to what has been called the "didactic tradition" of chemistry—a tradition whose roots lie firmly set in the seventeenth century.[1] Scholars have been aware of the ambiguous intentions of Paracelsian physicians who describe the preparation of medicaments for a long time. No matter how speculative and mystical their underlying philosophy of nature, when it came to describing remedies Paracelsian physicians remained largely unaffected by mystical jargon and magical allusions. In most instances, references to the preparation of medicines appeared as practical pharmaceutical recipes set aside from discussions of Paracelsus's medical cosmology. Just such a distinction between theory and practice affected the whole organization of one of the most widely consulted Paracelsian formularies of the early seventeenth century, Oswald Croll's *Basilica chymica* (1609).

To read Croll's text is to read what seems to be two books in one. Part of the volume is altogether practical and concerns the preparation of chemical remedies by various techniques, often by producing chemical reactions through the agency of mineral acids.[2] However, Croll devoted an even larger part of the text, including a long *Praefatio admonitoria* (Admonitory Preface) to theoretical discussions bearing on such themes as Paracelsian natural philosophy, the doctrine of signatures, the analogy between the macrocosm and microcosm, and the proper role of the hermetic physician. Depending upon which section one reads, Croll can be made to appear either as a practical chemical pharmacist, whose preparations continued to be listed in pharmacopoeias well into the nineteenth century,[3] or as one of the most mystical and speculative Paracelsian philosophers. Croll's own intent, however, as Owen Hannaway has skillfully shown, was certainly not to divide the two.[4]

[1] For a discussion of the didactic tradition see Owen Hannaway, *The Chemists and the Word: The Didactic Origins of Chemistry* (Baltimore and London: The Johns Hopkins University Press, 1975). Cf. Jan V. Golinski, "Chemistry in the Scientific Revolution: Problems of language and communication," in *Reappraisals of the Scientific Revolution*, ed. David C. Lindberg and Robert S. Westman (Cambridge: Cambridge University Press, 1990), pp. 367–396.

[2] Robert Multhauf, "Medical Chemistry and 'The Paracelsians'," *Bulletin of the History of Medicine* 28(1954):101–126. Also, Gerald Schröder, "Studien zur Geschichte der Chemiatrie," *Pharmazeutische Zeitung* 111(1966):1246–51.

[3] Gerald Schröder, *Die pharmazeutische-chemischen Produkte deutschen Apotheken im Zeitalter der Chemiatrie* (Bremen, 1957).

[4] Hannaway, *The Chemists and the Word* (n.1), chapters 1–3.

For Croll and other Paracelsians, the preparation of chemical remedies followed from a view of nature that assumed the existence of spiritual forces lying hidden in matter. These forces themselves could be manipulated by a practitioner who understood nature's inherent, magical powers. Medical and pharmaceutical knowledge required, therefore, an understanding of what had been concealed in creation. Nature possessed secrets and these were to be known only through revelation. But revelation could come about in two ways. Knowledge could be either mystically inspired, the so-called "light of grace," or arise indirectly as personal illumination through worldly experience, the "light of nature."[5] On this basis, that is, on the basis of epistemology, rests the distinction between approaches to nature that were and were not didactically influential. According to Owen Hannaway, who has done more than anyone else to define those distinctions, "knowledge for the Paracelsians was not a dialogue between experience and intellect motivated by reason: it arose from the action of the light of nature on the imagination to produce a comprehension of the powers and activities of the virtues of nature."[6] Skills in the laboratory and the techniques involved in the preparation of novel chemical remedies were not human inventions, but simply "externalized and controlled manifestations of the inherent powers of nature."[7] Since there was nothing to teach, methodologically speaking, Paracelsian chemical philosophy could not take part in a "didactic tradition." Insights into the forces of nature depended upon illumination of the imagination mediated through individual experience. Thus, from Hannaway's point of view, didactic chemistry could not develop out of Paracelsian chemical medicine by simply cutting away the mystical content of chemical philosophy. Instead, the didactic tradition depended upon a completely different ideology, one in which knowledge progressed as a "collective endeavor," and in which individual

[5] Concerning the light of grace and the light of nature see Kurt Goldammer, *Paracelsus: Natur und Offenbarung* (Hanover: Theodor Oppermann Verlag, 1953). *Idem*, "Lichtsymbolik in philosophischer Weltanschauung, Mystik und Theosophie vom 15. bis zum 17. Jahrhundert," *Studium Generale* 13(1960):677–682. Also, Kurt Goldammer (ed.), *Vom Licht der Natur und des Geistes* (Stuttgart: Philipp Reclam, 1979).

[6] Hannaway, *The Chemists and the Word* (n.1), p. 59.

[7] Hannaway, *The Chemists and the Word* (n.1), p. 59.

contributions to knowledge could be submitted to the examination of a community sharing an agreed upon and transmittable method of inquiry.[8]

Although Hannaway's distinctions make good sense at the level of epistemology, they do not account for the fact that Paracelsian chemical philosophy had an important place in the didactic chemical tradition despite its mystical components and its acceptance of divine illumination in understanding nature. Although Paracelsian philosophy was not epistemologically rational, that is, adhering to a transmittable method of inquiry, it was reasonable and very effective when considered empirically as laboratory pharmacy. This should not come as a surprise since what went by the name of Paracelsian philosophy and pharmacy was really formed out of quite distinct intellectual traditions.

Paracelsus advanced very little that was entirely new, either in terms of natural philosophy or pharmacy. The mystical philosophies of Renaissance Platonism and Hermeticism contributed, on the one hand, to the creation of an interconnected Paracelsian medical cosmology full of correspondences, sympathies, and astral emanations. But it was another tradition, one linked to the pharmaceutical preparations of the ancients and augmented by a knowledge of minerals and mineral compounds drawn from medieval alchemical texts, that was most responsible for the chemical medicines recorded by Paracelsian physicians. Paracelsian chemical cosmology made sense of the effects of medicaments the Paracelsians chose to call their own, but Paracelsian philosophy was not necessary to actually prepare them. From the Paracelsian point of view, pharmacy did indeed confirm philosophy. However, the two endeavors were nevertheless operationally distinct. As the emergence of non-Paracelsian iatrochemistry in the early seventeenth century suggests, knowledge of chemical medicines could be obtained through the didactic tradition.

What Paracelsus combined (Renaissance mysticism and medieval alchemy) could, of course, also be separated again. Some later editions of Croll's work, in fact, deemphasized its original speculative content. The English edition of 1670, for example, omitted the Admonitory Preface altogether.[9] The

[8] Hannaway, *The Chemists and the Word* (n.1), preface and pp. 152ff.

[9] *Royal and Practical Chymistry*. . . (London: Printed for John Starkey, 1670).

point is that although the reader of Paracelsian texts and pharmaceutical formularies needed to endure their mystical content, some of those same texts could still be useful tools of instruction. But what could make Paracelsian chemical philosophy didactically useful? In my view, an important element was space.[10]

Simply put, joining mystical philosophy with practical alchemical technique helped to create Paracelsian chemical philosophy. Making space between the two relieved Paracelsian chemical pharmacy of at least some of its mystical burden. Whereas the intellectual space of chemical pharmacy was still largely defined by the dimensions of Paracelsian natural philosophy, the visible exhibition of the supposed truth of that philosophy (the making of chemical medicines) required a different sort of space in which to operate. What was needed was a supporting physical environment, a workshop or laboratory, for instance. There the language in use depended less upon the "word," i.e., the language chosen to explicate nature within a philosophical milieu, than upon simple manual technique, i.e., the instrumental and practical language of laboratory demonstration. That sort of language, experiential rather than written, was didactically useful. And while students may have been encouraged to view it as manifestly linked with the secret language of nature, there was, in regard to the goals of laboratory activity, no necessity to do so. That is why Johannes Hartmann, the focus of this study, found it possible not only to edit the first edition of Croll's *Basilica*, with all its mystical content, but also to enlarge the practical parts of Croll's text in a later, annotated edition, and to employ parts of the volume as a didactic tool for the purpose of instructing students in his laboratory course in *chymiatria*. It is important not to be misunderstood here. To Hartmann, the recipes explained and duplicated by students in the laboratory served to declare the correctness of the vital philosophy he accepted. The epistemology of personal inspiration was still present in the labo-

[10] Concerning the relationship of physical spaces to the production of knowledge, especially of the experimental sort, see Steven Shapin and Simon Schaffer, *Leviathan and the Air-Pump: Hobbes, Boyle, and the Experimental Life* (Princeton: Princeton University Press, 1985); Owen Hannaway, "Laboratory Design and the Aim of Science: Andreas Libavius versus Tycho Brahe," *Isis*, 77(1986):585–610; and Steven Shapin, "The House of Experiment in Seventeenth-Century England," *Isis* 79(1988):373–404.

ratory, but it was not the focus of attention, because the language upon which it depended was not the language in use there. Nowhere in his diary of chemical instruction, in fact, does Hartmann specifically comment upon Paracelsian theory. In the contract struck between Hartmann and his students, an agreement that states precisely what each expects of the other, it was not the "word" that mattered. Rather, it was the hands-on doing of chemical pharmacy that counted.

PART ONE

Chymiatria at Marburg and its Theoretical Foundations

Didactic Pharmacy and Textbooks of Chemistry in the Seventeenth Century

The seventeenth century was, as has been frequently noticed, remarkably fertile in the production of practical chemical manuals and textbooks. Nearly all contained procedures, techniques, and recipes relevant to chemical pharmacy. Major chemical summaries whose purpose was clearly didactic appeared especially in the latter half of the century.[11] French chemical textbooks were particularly prominent. One of the most popular was Nicolas Le Fèvre's *Traicté de la Chymie* (Paris, 1660) which, although insisting that chemistry did not entirely consist of making remedies, nevertheless gave over substantial parts of itself to descriptions of chemical medicines. That was a pattern other chemical texts would follow, especially Christophe Glaser's *Traité de la Chymie* (1663), Johann Joachim Becher's *Oedipus chimicus* (1664), Nicolas Lemery's *Cours de Chymie* (1675),[12] and Michael Ettmüller's *Chimia rationalis ac experimentalis curiosa* (1684).

These later works made use of preparations found in Paracelsian formularies and were heavily influenced by discussions of applied chemistry included in technical-alchemical texts like Libavius's *Alchymia* (1597) and Rudolf Glauber's *Furni*

[11] For a nice summary see Lynn Thorndike, "Chemical Courses and Manuals," *A History of Magic and Experimental Science* (New York and London: Columbia University Press, 1964), vol. 8, Chap. 27. Also, Owen Hannaway, "Early University Courses in Chemistry," Ph.D. diss., The University of Glasgow, 1965.

[12] Lemery also published a synthesis of pharmaceutical manuals containing many of his own remedies in 1697, the *Pharmacopée universelle*.

novi philosophici (1648). By mid-century, laboratory courses joining chemistry and chemical pharmacy appeared in addition to didactic texts. At Paris, two Paracelsian court physicians, Turquet de Mayerne (1573–1655) and Jean Ribit, sieur de la Rivière (1571–1605), interceded on behalf of the royal almoner, Jean Beguin, in pursuing plans for constructing a laboratory and giving public lectures in chemistry and chemical medicine.[13] So that students would not be plagued by excessive note taking, Beguin privately published a laboratory manual destined to become one of the most frequently consulted chemical-pharmaceutical texts of the early seventeenth century.

Beguin's text, the *Tyrocinum chymicum* (1610), may have been touted as chemistry, but it was really pharmacy—albeit of a chemical sort. The context of the book is alchemical, and Beguin himself saw no problem in expropriating for his own use whole sections from Libavius's *Alchymia*. It was not, however, the transmutation of metals that concerned him. Instead, he concentrated upon obtaining medicaments from the purified subtle spirits of metals, gems, and plants. In a real sense, chemistry was pharmacy. In fact, the opening lines of the *Tyrocinum chymicum* defined chemistry as "the art of dissolving natural mixed bodies, of coagulating that which is dissolved, and preparing safer, more agreeable, and more healthful medicaments."[14] Chemists knew "the truth about the malignity of remedies." For, "things dug from the earth [*fossilia*], are plainly able to be reduced to that moderate nature [*ad eam mediocritatis naturam*], the whole being resolved into the parts making it up, and the malignant qualities removed." In this way chemists "admit into the innermost parts [*penetralia*] of their lives not a murderous enemy, but a friendly guest, not

[13] On Beguin and his chemical-pharmaceutical course at Paris see T.S. Patterson, "Jean Beguin and his Tyrocinium chymicum," *Annals of Science* 2(1937):243–298; A. Kent and O. Hannaway, "Some New Considerations on Beguin and Libavius," *Annals of Science* 16(1960):241–250.

[14] I have used Hartmann's edition: *In Johannis Beguini Regis Galliae Eleemosynarii Tyrocinium Chymicum Notae D. Johannis Hartmanni Olim editae a Christophoro Glückradt Phil et Medic. Doct.* in Hartmann, *Opera Omnia Medico-Chymica. . .*, ed. Conrado Johrenio, 7 vols. (Frankfurt am Main: Balthas. Christophori Wursti, 1684), 3: p. 5, col. 1. (Hereafter, *Opera Omnia*).

poisons, but *alexapharmaca* and an antidote against all diseases."[15]

As a laboratory manual, theory played no role at all in the *Tyrocinium*. Individual recipes, procedural definitions, the explanation of techniques, descriptions of vessels, and specific references to spirits, oils, liquid tinctures, balsams, extracts, and quintessences made up almost the whole of the volume. It was a practical handbook of chemical pharmacy and as such it enjoyed a popularity far beyond Beguin's Paris laboratory. A pirated edition appeared almost immediately, and a French translation of a revised text, *Les Élémens de Chymie*, was published in 1615. Three years later one of Beguin's pupils, Jeremias Barth, translated the text into Latin in an edition made larger by his own contributions. That edition, however, would have to contend with another, one composed in the same year by Johannes Hartmann, but not published until 1634. To judge by size alone, Hartmann's edition, which appeared under the pseudonym Christoph Glückradt, was the more attractive. It was twice as large as Beguin's original text, reflecting the addition of many of Hartmann's own notes, secrets, and medicinal recipes.

At Paris the teaching of chemical medicine continued after Beguin at the Jardin du Roi. This garden was founded in 1626, mostly at the urging of Paracelsian physicians, for the cultivation of medicinal plants. By 1640, the Jardin also served a pedagogic function, equipped with lecture halls and laboratories. A few years thereafter, the Jardin added a teaching position in chemistry and botany. The man chosen to fill that position, a transplanted Scotsman named William Davidson (c.1593–c.1669), was one of the king's physicians who was already teaching informal courses at Paris in chemical medicine.[16] By the time of his appointment, Davidson had written, for the benefit of students, his most important work: the *Philosophia pyrotechnica seu curriculus chymiatricus*.[17] In contrast to Beguin's *Tyrocinium*, the *Philosophia pyrotechnica*

[15] *Tyrocinium Chymicum* (n.14), in *Opera Omnia*, 3:p. 6, col. 2.

[16] John Read, "William Davidson of Aberdeen: The First British Professor of Chemistry," *Ambix* 9(1961):70–101. Cf. Rio Howard, *La bibliothèque et le laboratoire de Guy La Brosse au Jardin des Plantes à Paris*, Histoire et civilisation du livre, 13 (Geneva: Droz, 1983).

[17] The first and second parts of this work (published in 1635) were actually preceded by parts three and four, which were published in 1633.

included much that was metaphysical and philosophical. A review of practical operations in the making of chemical medicines was wedged into the text as a concluding fourth part. However, with the publication of a greatly expanded and rearranged French translation, *Les Élémens de la Philosophie de l'Art de Feu ou Chemie* (1651), Davidson began to turn more directly to the practical details of individual medicinal preparations from plants, animals, and minerals.

Although teachers of chemical medicine, neither Beguin nor Davidson could claim a position within the university. There were, however, several at this time who did make inroads into the academic environment. One was Zacharias Brendel (1592–1638) who offered a public lecture course in the making of chemical medicaments at the University of Jena around 1630.[18] The year following Brendel's death, a fellow Jena professor who had taught anatomy, surgery, botany, and medical chemistry, Werner Rolfinck (1599–1673), continued chemical instruction. At that time he acquired the more specific title of *Director exerciti chymici* (director of chemical exercises).[19] There were others, like Johann Daniel Mylius, G. Horst, and L. Jungermann at the University of Giessen, who could also be counted as being involved in teaching chemical pharmacy in some capacity. However, in terms of establishing chemical pharmacy as an independent discipline within the university curriculum, no appointment equals in significance the naming of Johannes Hartmann to the position of *Professor publicus chymiatriae* at the University of Marburg in 1609. To understand what led up to that appointment we must first sketch Hartmann's early career both at court and at the university. Thereafter we can look more specifically both at the philosophical and the practical content of the discipline he represented.

Hartmann's Career to 1609

For Hartmann, the road to the laboratory of chemical medicine in Marburg began in Kassel, at the court of the univer-

[18] The text that Brendel published for his course was called *Chimia in artis formam redacta* (Jena, 1630).

[19] Rolfinck published his own chemical text using Brendel's title: *Chimia in artis formam redacta, sex libris comprehensa* (Jena, 1661).

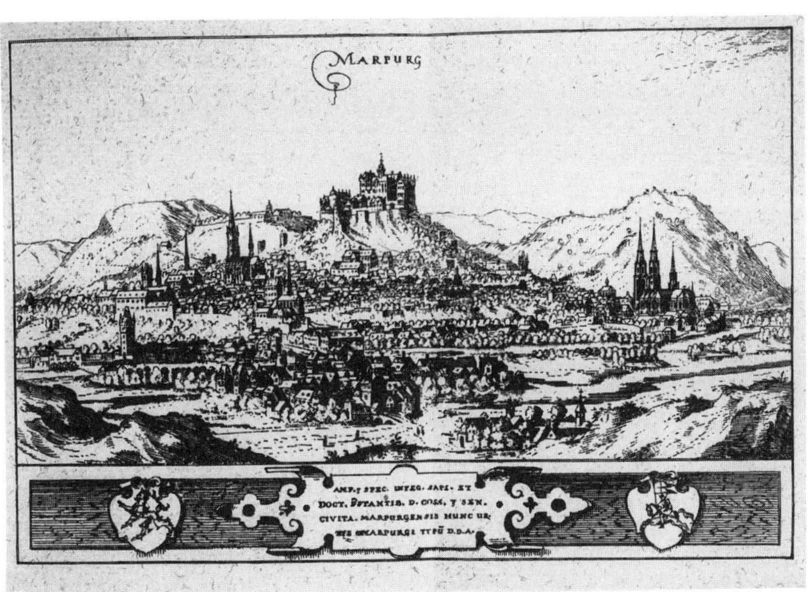

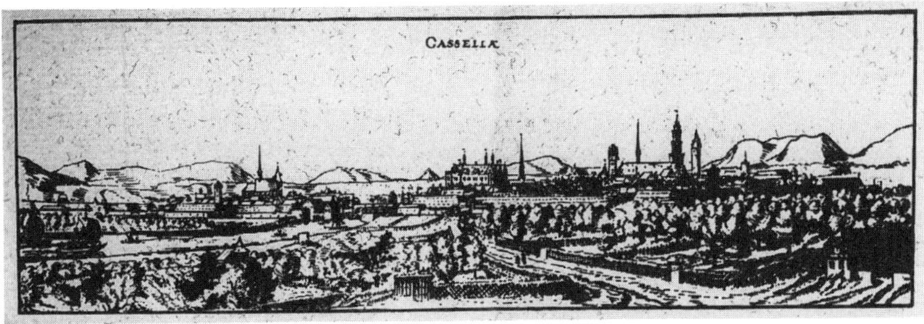

Marburg and Kassel around the time of Hartmann's appointment as Professor publicus chymiatriae, *from Wilhelm Dilich,* Hessische Chronica *(1605).*

sity's protector, the Landgrave Moritz of Hesse (1572–1632).[20] It was there that he appeared in the early 1590s after completing studies, primarily in mathematics, at several universities, most recently at the University of Wittenberg.[21] The court needed a mathematician and Hartmann got the job. But the residence in Kassel was to be only temporary. With the death of the Marburg professor of mathematics, Victorin Schönfeld, a position in the university's faculty of arts opened and Hartmann, with Moritz's consent, was chosen to fill it. But teaching at Marburg did not preclude continued involvement with the court in Kassel. Hartmann remained a court consultant and, in 1598, left the university on a two-year leave-of-absence to help Moritz with an editorial project aimed at publishing the optical works of Friedrich Risner (d. 1580) and to teach in the Landgrave's court school.

What Hartmann experienced during his second stay at court can only be guessed. At that time he surely came to know two recently appointed court physicians, Hermann Wolf (c.1562–1620) and Jacob Mosanus (1564–1616). Both were busy making and testing chemical medicaments for the Landgrave and his family, and Hartmann would have noticed that their pharmacological activity on behalf of the court corresponded to a

[20] I have sketched the relationship of Hartmann and the Kassel court in "Court Authority and Chemical Medicine: Moritz of Hessen, Johannes Hartmann, and the Origin of Academic Chemiatria," *Bulletin of the History of Medicine* 63(1989):225–246.

[21] Information regarding Hartmann's life begins with Theophilus Newberger, ed., *Auss dem CXXI Psalm Davids, als dess weiland, Ehrnvesten . . . Herrn Johannis Hartmanni, . . . Verbliechener Leichnam am 11. Decembris dess 1631 Jahrs in seine Ruhstatte in der Haupt: Kirche . . . gesetzet worden, bey ansehenlicher volckreicher versamblung, gezeigt und erklaret, auch nun mehr auff begeren zum Truck verfertigt, durch Theophilium Newbergern* (Cassel: Johann Saurn, 1632). More recent references include Th. Kunzmann, "Der Webersohn Hartmann von Amberg," *Bayerische Heimat* 22(1941):125–26; Rudolf Schmitz and Adolf Winckelmann, "Johann Hartmann (1568–1631), 'Doctor Medicus et Chymiatriae Professor Publicus,' Eine Biographisches Skizze," *Pharmazeutische Zeitung* 111(1966):1233–41; W. Hubicki, "Uczniowie z Polski na Studiach Chymiatrii w Marburga w Latach 1609–1620," *Studia i Materialy z Dziejów Nauki Polskiej* 12(1968):79–103. Also, Rudolf Schmitz, *Die Naturwissenschaften an der Philipps-Universität Marburg* (Marburg: N.G. Elwert, 1978), pp. 193–202; *idem*, "Die Universität Kassel und ihre Beziehung zu Pharmazie und Chemie," *Pharmazeutische Zeitung* 104(1959):1413–17; *idem*, "Der Apotheker im Wandel der Jahrhunderte," *Pharmazeutische Zeitung* 102(1957):1323–27.

change in the interests of the prince himself. Since the time of their first meeting Moritz had become captivated by the study of occult philosophy, especially in relation to alchemy, and was well on his way to amassing an extensive collection of alchemical, Cabbalistic, and Paracelsian manuscripts, and to fashioning a court circle of alchemical and medical adepts.[22] I have suggested elsewhere that changes in the direction of court patronage at Kassel were among the factors most responsible for changes in Hartmann's own disciplinary focus.[23] Chances to enjoy the favor of the court were slim if one's talents were defined solely in terms of mathematics. But Hartmann himself harbored other interests that could lead to real advancement, if given a formal footing. Thus, following his return to Marburg, he began reading for a medical degree, which he received in 1606. He also began a brief correspondence with the French Paracelsian, Joseph Duchesne (Quercetanus)(c. 1544–1609). In 1604, when Duchesne visited Kassel and revealed there the preparation of a great number of chemical remedies, Hartmann was one of those present at a temporary laboratory set up for the demonstrations. At the same time Hartmann sought out and read the alchemical texts of Basil Valentine and corresponded with Johann Thölde, then admired as the editor of Basilian writings, but now generally regarded as having actually composed them himself.[24] The pharmaceutical uses of antimony described by Basil particularly impressed Hartmann and he made no secret thereafter of his laboratory successes. In letters to Duchesne he claimed to have extracted Basil's universal medicament, the "Stone of Fire," and confided also that he had made other medicines involving antimony and mercury.[25]

In the three years between 1606 and 1609 Hartmann held a joint appointment at Marburg as professor of mathematics and medicine. That appointment was tied to others at the university designed to carry the intellectual ideals of the Kassel court into the Marburg curriculum. Court ideology, embracing

[22] Bruce T. Moran, "Privilege, Communication, and Chemiatry: The Hermetic-Alchemical Circle of Moritz of Hessen-Kassel," *Ambix* 32(1985):110–126.

[23] Moran, "Court Authority and Chemical Medicine," (n.20), *passim*.

[24] Hans Gerhard Lenz, "Johann Thölde: ein Paracelsist und 'Chymicus' und seine Beziehung zu Landgraf Moritz von Hessen-Kassel," Ph.D. diss., University of Marburg, 1981, pp. 53–57.

[25] Staats- und Universitätsbibliothek, Hamburg Sup. ep. (4°)30, 7r-9r.

a view of nature interwoven with correspondences, signatures, and astral influences, found its way into various university faculties via a new group of professors whose members espoused principles of Neoplatonic and Paracelsian natural philosophy. In 1606, Raphael Eglinus (1559–1622), a Swiss Calvinist known for his alchemical enthusiasm and for his association with the Italian hermeticist Giordano Bruno, was appointed to the theological faculty. Two years later Rudolf Goclenius the younger (1572–1621), an adherent to principles of correspondence and natural sympathies and an advocate of the Paracelsian weapon salve, gained the chair of physics and was soon thereafter appointed to professorships in medicine (1611) and mathematics (1613). The medical professor Heinrich Ellenberger (c.1570–1624), who left the university in 1607, officially for religious reasons, also held to a hermetic medical philosophy.[26] Later, another of Moritz's appointees, Johannes Combach, added to the depth of mystical and occult traditions represented among the Marburg faculty.

At first glance, Hartmann appears as simply one of many to make his way at the university by reflecting the values of his patron at the Kassel court. Yet he enjoyed a special place. More than anyone else within the faculty of medicine, he combined an understanding of Hermetic/Paracelsian cosmology with an acquired skill in practical laboratory technique. In 1607, that practical knowledge led to an ill-fated alchemical contract with a Herborn schoolmaster named Heinrich Dauber. Dauber was to supply the *materia* and Hartmann the laboratory space and expertise necessary for preparing the Philosophers' Stone. Each ultimately blamed the other for the project's failure; but it was Dauber who later brought the affair to the attention of the landgrave, claiming that Hartmann may have actually only feigned the negative results so as to keep the powerful transmuting agent for himself.[27] Alchemical failures aside, Moritz valued Hartmann's alchemical insights, especially as they related to making chemical medicines and, in 1608, enthusiastically received a suggestion from Hartmann for founding a

[26] Andreas Libavius refers to Ellenberger as *Medicus Hermeticus Hassiae* (i.e., hermetic physician of Hesse). *Syntagmatis arcanorum chymicorum. . .*(Frankfurt am Main: Nicolaus Hoffmannus, 1613), p. 246.

[27] Murhardsche Bibliothek der Stadt Kassel, 2° MS Chem 19, 1: 90r-v. Hereafter Murhardsche Bibliothek.

MAURITIUS DEI GRATIA HASSIÆ LANDGRAVIUS: CATTIMELIBOCI: DECII: ZIGENHAIN: ET NIDDÆ COMES:
Ætatis suæ 44
Anno 1616
Consilio et Virtute

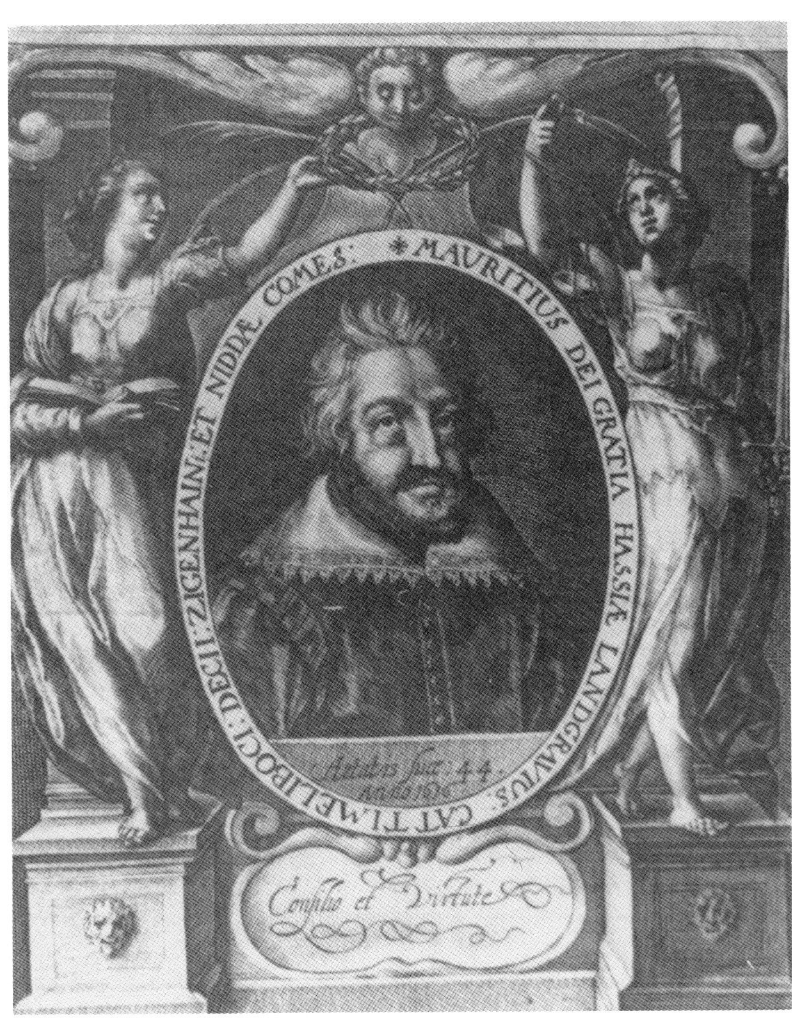

Crispin van de Passe, Moritz of Hessen *(1616).*

collegium chymicum at Marburg. The idea gained the encouragement of Moritz's court physicians, Wolf and Mosanus, and led the prince, in the following year, to announce the creation of a new course at Marburg to be taught within the medical school. The new subject was to be based upon both reading and practical laboratory exercises, by means of which students would be instructed in the preparation of chemical medicines. Hartmann possessed the philosophical and practical skills that the discipline required. More important, those skills were counted as abilities worthy of court patronage. For these reasons Moritz chose to invest Hartmann with a new university role and a new title—*Professor publicus chymiatriae.*

Paracelsian physicians were well established at many central European courts, but nowhere other than at Marburg had anyone gained official entrance into university circles for the purpose of teaching chemical medicine. In France, well known Paracelsians like Joseph Duchesne and Theodore Mayerne, although admitted into the circle of physicians surrounding the French king Henri IV, struggled in vain to convince the Paris medical faculty of the value of teaching spagyric medicine. A book written by Duchesne in 1604, *Ad veritatem hermeticae medicinae ex Hippocratis veterumque decretis ac therapeusi*, argued that Paracelsian and traditional Hippocratic and Galenic studies were in fact compatible and of equal importance for medical students. The book, however, found few academic supporters. Instead, another book appeared written by a spokesman of the Paris medical faculty, Jean Riolan, which included an attack upon the Paracelsians at the king's court. Thereafter, polemical salvos erupted from both sides with the battleground extending finally far beyond the borders of France. Even Andreas Libavius (1540–1616), whom we shall meet again as a bitter opponent of Paracelsian philosophy, entered the debate to defend the legitimacy of chemistry in medicine.[28]

Events at Paris were well known both at the Kassel court and at the University of Marburg. Moritz, in fact, kept part of the original debate between Duchesne and Riolan in his private

[28] On the controversy at Paris see Hugh Trevor-Roper, "The Paracelsian Movement," *Renaissance Essays* (Chicago: University of Chicago Press, 1985), pp. 149–99.

chemical library. To the Kassel prince, the Paris affair must have appeared as a dramatic and much publicized failure among chemical physicians in France to secure a place for themselves within the university. But what had failed in Paris due to the opposition of the medical faculty might be made to succeed at Marburg by direct command of the university's *Landesherr*. In Hesse, where the prince's control of university affairs was direct and absolute, a place for the study of *chymiatria*, requiring room within the medical faculty for a new set of ideas and a new sort of physical environment (a laboratory), could be created by court decree. Yet as we shall see, while the creation of both spaces, intellectual and physical, depended upon the will of the prince, the discipline's professor, Johannes Hartmann, defined their limits and controlled what was expected of those crossing their threshold.

Hartmann's Entrance Oration and the Definition of *Chymiatria*

As expected of every newly appointed professor, Hartmann prepared an hour-long public oration that he delivered to an audience of students, faculty, and university dignitaries on the fourth of April, 1609.[29] Most in attendance would have known already that Hartmann's medical philosophy was not the traditional Galenic sort. Thus, few would have been surprised by Hartmann's reference to himself in the title of his address as *philosophus, sive naturae consultus medicus* (philosopher, or experienced physician of nature). He might just as well have chosen to describe himself as "Paracelsian practitioner and disciple of hermetic philosophy." The effect would have been the same.

In writing the inaugural address, Hartmann was keenly aware that *chymiatria* might be seen by some as an unwelcome addition to the medical curriculum at Marburg. Thus he began by reminding fellow professors that both the new discipline and his own position as *Professor publicus chymiatricae* had come into being through the wisdom and authority of the university's protector, the Landgrave Moritz of Hesse. Only then,

[29] *Joh. Hartmanni, M.D. In Academia Marburgensi Chymiatriae designat Profess. Philosophus sive Naturae Consultus Medicus: Oratione Publice ab ipso Propositus, IV Calend. Aprilis, Anno MDCIX*, in Hartmann, *Opera Omnia*, 4: pp. 3–19.

having established the legitimacy of his own view of medicine on the basis of court authority, did Hartmann insist that *chymia* (chemistry) be recognized as part of the liberal arts and turn to a defense of chemical pharmacy as an essential component of medical instruction. The result of the combination of chemistry and medicine, he argued, would be a new type of medical professional—one trained in *chymiatria*—thus combining Hippocratic medicine with Paracelsian pharmacy, so as to become a *naturae consultus medicus* like himself.[30]

It is a mark of Hartmann's own rhetorical skill that he could emphasize both chemistry's antiquity and its German roots as signs of its importance to human knowledge. Chemistry, he argued, had flourished among the ancients and had been counted among the most prized of all the arts by wise men, kings, and princes alike. By means of both chemistry and medicine ancient physicians became greatly skilled in the art of healing. Nevertheless, the world's perverse ingratitude for such a heavenly gift had been responsible for its neglect until:

> in the days of our fathers it happened that the barbarous and rustic Germans were inspired with the most kind breath of divine mercy and . . . the best examples of all the liberal arts began to be scattered like seeds. In the same way, our science could not be hidden any longer, but . . . came to be admired and cultivated again. Nor could it remain contained within the hiding places of monks . . . but burst through monastic walls and far and wide attached itself to the company of physicians.[31]

Chemistry's roots may have been both ancient and Germanic, but they were also non-academic. Some would insist, Hartmann knew, that chemistry was a lowly profession, the sordid business of barbers and servants. But those individuals would never know the true perfection of medicine, nor could they ever claim that their grasp of the liberal arts was complete.

> So why do we hesitate to grant deserved honors and the greatest dignity to that art without whose escort medicine has no, or at best has very little, majesty? Do we hesitate to raise this thing . . . that is [as some would claim] steeped in the filth of an unfit crowd and place it among the purple-clad faculties of Academia? But what am I doing? Why do I torture myself with

[30] As we shall see, Hartmann's eclectic approach to medicine was much influenced by Peter Severinus's *Idea medicinae philosophicae* (1571). For an in depth study of Severinus's work, see Jole Shackelford,"Paracelsianism in Denmark and Norway in the 16th and 17th Centuries," Ph.D. diss., University of Wisconsin, 1989, Chap. 2.

[31] *Oratione publice* (n.29), in *Opera Omnia*, 4:p. 6, col. 1.

empty complaints and vain cares? Why this despair? A remedy for this disease has been found . . . chemistry has been accepted [into the university] . . . by the courageous prince Moritz, our most kind *nutricus*. His wise counsel has seen to it that *chymiatria* will be practiced and taught publicly from the clearest springs of Hermetic and Hippocratic philosophy.[32]

Hartmann knew of the problems that the French Paracelsian Joseph Duchesne had endured at the hands of the Paris faculty of medicine. Thus he next laments that "even now there are not a few who, intoxicated, as if by a draught from the cup of Circe . . . would rather wander . . . in the thickest fog than to reason with the sober few." Such are the "Parisian doctors" who by attacking those who had turned to *chymiatria*, attempted "to proscribe God from the limits of the earth, and then to outlaw nature herself from the bosom of the entire university."[33]

Clearly, Hartmann, like Moritz, saw something succeeding at Marburg that had failed at Paris. Let the Parisian doctors publish their assaults on those who had turned away from "the monstrous failings of ordinary medicine." At Marburg there would be nurtured a more advanced sort of medical man, the *naturae consultus medicus*, that is, "the prudent man practiced in influencing nature" (*virum prudentem movendi naturam peritum*).[34] The Marburg *medicus* would learn not from precepts but by practice. He would be experienced in the laboratory, know how to make useful medicines, and understand what features from Hippocrates and Paracelsus should be combined to join the art of healing with effective pharmacy. Of course, the *naturae consultus medicus* would also comprehend the intimate harmonies of the universe, and thus understand the analogous relationship between man (the microcosm) and the macrocosm.

What is in the republic of the human body that has not itself been revealed in the greater ordering of the whole universe? What is in the miraculous structure of the world that man does not carry around in his own prison [*in ergastulo suo*]? For from nothing [comes] everything, and from everything [comes] man, clearly the ultimate creation by divine *Thechnurgema*. Man embraces everything in himself, and he himself bears all things in himself . . . He was made from the world and embraces the world in

[32] *Oratione publice* (n.29), in *Opera Omnia*, 4:p. 6, col. 1.
[33] *Oratione publice* (n.29), in *Opera Omnia*, 4:p. 7, col. 1.
[34] *Oratione publice* (n.29), in *Opera Omnia*, 4:p. 7, cols. 1 and 2.

himself and [thus] is embraced by the world. Therefore the great world harmonizes with the small by the shortest chain of unity and necessity. This is the reason the wisest of the ancients called man microcosm . . . [for] . . . in man there is the creator and the created universe.[35]

The task of the Marburg student of medicine and *chymiatria* is thus to become skilled in the study of the entire universe and to contemplate its harmonies. He must dwell, says Hartmann, within the whole world, fly over its seas, and burst through the ramparts of the heavens, collecting the motions and numbers of the stars and planets, arranging the elements, and seeking out the laws of generation and transplantation.[36] Then he will know "that the heavens, stars, and all airy, aquatic, and terrestrial things are lodged in man," that "lightening, thunder, hail, rain, heat, cold, and dryness in the external world are, in the invisible world of man, fevers, epilepsies, hydropsy, catarrh, paralyses, and apoplexies."[37]

Most of all, however, the *naturae consultus medicus* must be a physician-chemist (*medicus-chemicus*). The perfection of medicine depends upon an understanding of *chymia*. Thus the physician must inevitably be skilled in the theory and practice of alchemy. In Hartmann's view "the perfect *naturae consultus medicus* cannot be cut off from alchemy. For this one lamp of Diana has revealed more than [the learning of] all the vulgar physicians combined."[38] Among these, Hartmann quite clearly wants to include Galen and his followers, who knew nothing of the alchemical art. Hippocrates, on the other hand, knew that medicaments were made by separation and this is what the physician skilled in nature must also learn by a marriage of Vulcan and Pallas (i.e., fire and wisdom). In the end, then, *chymiatria* is really the fruit of a *nov-antiqua medicina*, a new-old medicine linking the preparations of medicines derived from Paracelsus and the chemists with the methods of Hippocratic healing. Knowing these things, the *naturae consultus medicus* influences nature by means of nature, examines the secrets of things through the service of the fire, and considers the world in the world of man.[39]

[35] *Oratione publice* (n.29), in *Opera Omnia*, 4:p. 9, col. 2.

[36] *Oratione publice* (n.29), in *Opera Omnia*, 4:p. 9, col. 1. On the notions of generation and transplantation as described by Peter Severinus, see Shackelford, "Paracelsianism in Denmark and Norway" (n.30), pp. 98–102.

[37] *Oratione publice* (n.29), in *Opera Omnia*, 4:p. 10, col. 1.

[38] *Oratione publice* (n.29), in *Opera Omnia*, 4:p. 10, col. 2.

[39] *Oratione publice* (n.29), in *Opera Omnia*, 4:p. 13, cols 1 and 2.

What reaction Hartmann's oration received from within the Marburg medical faculty is unknown. Since hermetic philosophers and Paracelsian physicians had already frequented the university, the address may not have caused much of a stir. It was not until 1613 that Hartmann got around to publishing the oration, adding to it a number of chemical-medical disputations written mostly under his direction. For our purposes, however, it is the preface of the published inaugural that is most interesting. There, in a subdued yet bitter way, Hartmann alludes to what he sees as a vicious assault recently launched upon him and his medical philosophy by an unnamed critic.

There are those, he says, who think they will appear learned if they accuse others of being unlearned. Nevertheless, Hartmann writes, "no matter how much a certain great *eclogarius* of chemical secrets has lately spewed out poisonous remarks against me, I do not judge it to be so important as perhaps the author desires of me."[40] In fact, Hartmann claims to have never done anything but praise his attacker's alchemical teachings and, in fact, to have openly commended them to his students. But there were certain things, especially what had been written about mercury and the Philosophers' Stone, that had been published, Hartmann contends, "with foolish judgment." He continues:

> These things I have discussed privately with friends, both personally and in letters, and have often detested his careless inattention to proper chemical elaboration . . . And so, as I have always publicly and privately proclaimed his legitimate understanding of alchemy, I have refuted the remaining sophisms in the liberal manner afforded by amicable conversation and letters among friends, that is, discreetly and never *kataphorikos* [i.e., openly]. But why then was I so frivolously and violently attacked in print? What was the great crime for which I should be so exposed to ridicule? God as my witness, nothing seemed more unreasonable. That rattle of Archytas seemed to have had nothing else in mind, a mind born to calumny as it turns out, than to make use of the opportunity to attack my name, to grab it with his . . . teeth . . . and to trample it underfoot as much as he could.[41]

The attack clearly angered Hartmann, and while proclaiming that he would not respond in kind by way of a verbal assault, Hartmann did actually plan a response. The publication of his inaugural was part of that response. The preface called upon

[40] *Oratione publice* (n.29), *Opera Omnia*, 4:pp. 3–4.
[41] *Oratione publice* (n.29), *Opera Omnia*, 4:p. 4.

students of hermetic medicine to come to the aid of their wounded teacher. By entering his *laboratorium chemico-medicum* and learning from him the preparation of chemical medicines they would help heal the terrible bite made by his assailant.

You medical novices, whoever you are, you who wish to be taught medicine's cure for the bite of the sycophant, come and stand with me. Just as physicians prescribe human excrement [a Paracelsian remedy] for a bite made by a man, apply a squared plaster to my slanderer . . . lest he bite forever.[42]

Who was the unnamed critic by whom Hartmann felt so unjustly abused? Everything points to one man, to one of the best known and most respected chemists of the late sixteenth and early seventeenth centuries, the Coburg chemist, physician, and pedagogue, Andreas Libavius (1540–1616). The bite that Hartmann considered so venomous had almost certainly been caused by one of Libavius's texts, his *Appendix necessaria syntagmatis arcanorum chymicorum* (Frankfurt, 1615).[43] This was an enormous volume composed of lengthy attacks aimed mostly at Paracelsian and Hermetic authors. Among those to be polemically skewered were Henning Scheunemann and Oswald Croll (c. 1560–1609).[44] One whole section, however, two hundred and sixty-one pages, was reserved for the Danish Paracelsian, Petrus Severinus (1542–1602), and for the Severinian "vital philosophy" that had been adopted by the Marburg professor and physician, Johannes Hartmann.

The book to which these polemics were attached, Libavius's *Syntagmatis arcanorum chymicorum*, had been published already in 1613.[45] Although the pieces to appear in the "Appendix" were not published until 1615, it is quite likely that they already existed and had possibly circulated in some form when

[42] *Oratione publice* (n.29), in *Opera Omnia*, 4:p. 4.

[43] *D.O.M.A. Appendix necessaria Syntagmatis Arcanorum Chymicorum Andreae Libavii M.D.P.C. Halli-Saxonis illustris Gymnasii apud Corburgenses Directoris, Professoris publ. et Medici Chymici-practici. In Qua Praeter Arcanorum Nonnullorum expositionem et illustrationem, quorundam item Medicorum Hermeticorum, et mysteriorum descriptionem, continentur defensiones genuinae* . . . (Frankfurt, 1615).

[44] For a discussion of the polemics, especially as they relate to Oswald Croll, see Owen Hannaway, *The Chemists and the Word* (n.1), Chapter 5.

[45] *D.O.M.A. Syntagmatis Arcanorum Chymicorum, ex Optimis Autoribus Scriptis, impressis, experientiaque artifice collectorum* . . . (Frankfurt am Main: Nicolaus Hoffmannus, 1613).

the main work first appeared. Hartmann, writing in 1613, was already able to refer to the attack upon him as being mounted as part of a collection (*eclogarius*) of writings. The alchemical teachings that he had praised and recommended to students were probably those of Libavius's didactic text of chemical *praxis*, the *Alchymia* (Frankfurt, 1597). But Hartmann had not praised everything and admits that he had also written frankly of his criticisms in private letters. At the beginning of his critique of Severinus and Hartmann, Libavius also writes of letters, especially concerning one from Hartmann to the son of Martin Ruland, as a result of which their relationship had gone sour.

Specifically, Libavius notes that he and Hartmann had been friends in Marburg in 1601. However, after Hartmann had been named professor of mathematics and had then studied *chymiatria*, he had written to Ruland saying that Libavius was so unskilled in his chemical guidance that he had begun to cause shame and had prostituted himself before the whole world. The problem was that what Hartmann explained as a private letter among friends, Libavius considered to be a public document. What Hartmann described as comments set in "the liberal manner afforded by amicable conversation," Libavius viewed as being broadcast "in the clear light of the imperial court," making it difficult for the *studia Libaviana* to be recommended there. It was a case of lost patronage and Libavius held Hartmann responsible. He believed that Hartmann's letter, which was sent on to him by Ruland, was laced with treachery. Possibly Hartmann himself had ambitions at the imperial court and wished to undercut his own chances. Also deceitful from Libavius's point of view was the way that Hartmann, after criticizing chemical procedures openly and honestly sent to him, especially those concerned with the elaboration of mercury, had withheld from him his own process for mercury's precipitation.[46]

It is not difficult to find the source of the problems that developed between Hartmann and Libavius. Within the context of alchemical patronage at court, advancing one's own ideas often

[46] *D.O.M.A. De philosophia vivente seu vitali Paracelsi iuxta P. Severinum Danum ex repetitione I. Hartmanni chymiatri Marburgensis. Praefatio ad I. Hartmanni.* This narrative is collected together with polemics aimed at Croll and the Rosicrucians in a special section of the *Appendix necessaria syntagmatis arcanorum chymicorum* (1615) beginning with its own title page: *D.O.M.A. Examen philosophiae novae, quae veteri abrogandae opponitur* . . . (Frankfurt am Main: Petrus Kopffius, 1615).

meant attacking other claims. Hartmann understood the patronage game far better than Libavius. Between physicians and chemists there might exist a considerable degree of openness and sharing of ideas; but when it came to selling those ideas to the court a different set of expectations needed to be addressed. Patronage, especially alchemical-pharmaceutical patronage, often depended upon convincing the prince that one had privileged information to offer. There were numerous ways in which one might promote the essential secrecy of alchemical and pharmaceutical ideas. One might claim special insight through revelation, or argue, as apparently Hartmann did, that one's own work had advanced further than others—that potential competitors were misinformed or outright swindlers. In this sense, the relationship between Hartmann and Libavius appears as a curious mixture of secrecy, openness, acknowledged friendship, and bitter hatred. Yet none of this was in the least bit unusual. From the point of view of pursuing and protecting favor at court, one might almost have predicted a falling out between the two in that instant when one began to suspect the other of becoming a potential rival.

Hartmann's Vital Philosophy

Libavius's attack was an attempt to discredit a certain type of medical philosophy that increasingly had gained preference within court circles. In mounting it, he concentrated especially upon the notion of a "vital philosophy" that became the focus of a small tract attributed to Hartmann titled *Introductio in vitalem philosophiam.*[47] Who actually wrote the text is unclear. It survives in Hartmann's *Opera,* published in 1684; but by then it had already appeared, also posthumously, as the work of Johann Ernst Burggrav, published at Frankfurt in 1623. Whatever the origins of the text, there is enough connection to Hartmann to be safe in viewing it as generally reflecting the philosophical foundations of his medical practice and chemical preparations. For that reason, we ought to give

[47] *Introductio in Vitalem Philosophiam cui cohaeret omnium morborum astralium et materialium seu, morborum omnium, elementatorum et haereditariorum ex libro naturae, codice philosophicae et medicae veritatis, additis veterum placitis, Hippocratis, Galeni, Celsi, aliorum, Eplicatio atque Curatio* . . . in Hartmann, *Opera Omnia*, 7: pp. 1–61.

some attention to its contents before setting out to examine Libavius's hostile reaction to the philosophy it described.

At the heart of the little treatise are two often interrelated intellectual traditions: Paracelsian natural philosophy (itself based largely upon the Platonic thinking of the Renaissance) and hermetic alchemy. The book is an "introduction" and the author makes little claim to novelty. He relies upon already familiar notions linked to the works of Paracelsus and Paracelsian writers like Duchesne, Oswald Croll, and especially, Petrus Severinus. Like these, he too argues that there is one principle underlying all true philosophy, astronomy, medicine, and alchemy. Astronomers and magicians call it the invisible sun, philosophers and physicians refer to it as first matter (*primam materiam*), and physio-chemists call it the simple root of minerals (*radicem mineralium simplicem*). Whatever its name, it is the source of life and activity in all things and is therefore the universal vital principle. It is this principle that contains the characteristics and qualities of every existing species, and the text likens it to "the sphere of the Pythagoreans, equally diffused through all parts of the world, whose center is in our soul."[48] This vital principle or natural living fire is the seed of all generation and of all occult properties. It is the *leo viridis* of the physio-chemists, filling everything, connecting the soul to the world, and containing in itself all virtues.[49]

As with most Paracelsian works, this one agrees that all things are composed of soul (*anima*), spirit, and body. The essence of soul it equates with the vital principle of things, calling this principle an innate mummy, radical humor, or flower of the soul. It is the intermediary between spirit and body—that which "joins, couples, and unites diverse things and which combines them into one substance."[50]

Spirit, body, and soul first appear as part of a threefold unfolding or separation at the time of creation. From a pre-existing *ens primum creatum catholigum* are separated three principles: *coelum*, *spiritus mundi*, and *medium*. From *coe-*

[48] *Introductio in vitalem philosophiam* (n.47), in *Opera Omnia*, 7:p. 2, col. 2.

[49] *Introductio in vitalem philosophiam* (n.47), in *Opera Omnia*, 7:pp. 4, col. 1—5, col. 1.

[50] *Introductio in vitalem philosophiam* (n.47), in *Opera Omnia*, 7:pp. 7, col. 1—9, col. 1.

lum arose the *ruch elohim*, which the text defines as the spirit of God dwelling in water. From the *spiritus mundi*, thought of as a corporeal spirit permeating all things, arose the *anima mundi*, the blessed viridity that itself produces *leo viridis*. From *medium* (that which "is not body, but indeed soul, nor soul but actually body, joining two extremes") arose *forma*, that which gives being to things and which is their effective agent.[51]

Coinciding with the threefold origin of the universe, the *Introductio* thereafter identifies three things as necessary for any sort of generation. There must first be the elements, two of which are spiritual (fire and air) and two corporeal (water and earth), but each viewed in the Paracelsian sense, that is, as the matrices of things born into the world.[52] As a second necessity the writer refers to what he calls, following Severinus, either seeds, the first water, anima, or astra. These, he says, are the chains of the visible and invisible and contain in themselves the laws of motion and generation. The third essential ingredient of generation he defines as the principles of bodies, namely sulphur, salt, and mercury. These provide properties to things and produce in them their particular actions.[53]

Discussing generation is an important prelude to the text's real focus, the nature and cure of disease. Here it follows Paracelsus in assuming the existence of an *ens veneni*, one of five essences of disease discussed by Paracelsus in his *Volumen medicinae paramirum* (c. 1520).[54] An *ens* is that which has the power to govern, to transmute, or to influence bodies. Thus the *ens veneni* exists as one of the essences of creation. As with other essences, it too is transmitted by the stars as *astra* or seeds producing its fruit (physical disease) when generated in the elementary matrix of water and earth. Nothing in all of nature, says the author (following Paracelsus's description in

[51] *Introductio in vitalem philosophiam* (n.47), in *Opera Omnia*, 7:p. 10.

[52] This two-fold division of the elements into an upper and lower pair is a prominent feature of Severinus's treatment of the elements. See Shackelford, "Paracelsianism in Denmark and Norway" (n.30), p. 86.

[53] *Introductio in vitalem philosophiam* (n.47), in *Opera Omnia*, 7:p. 10, cols. 1 and 2.

[54] *Volumen Medicinae Paramirum of Theophrastus von Hohenheim called Paracelsus*, trans. Kurt F. Leidecker (Baltimore: The Johns Hopkins Press, 1949).

the *Chirurgia majore*), exists apart from this essence. Transmitted by the stars, the *ens veneni* enters animals, vegetables, and minerals. In all food, therefore, there is present the *ens veneni* which, if not correctly separated in the stomach, is the cause of most severe illnesses.[55]

Thus, all species of poisons that produce fruits in the inferior world are contained equally in the stars. "If, indeed," the author writes, "all the properties and *astra* of the heavens and the earth are contained in man, and because of this man is called microcosmos, even Libavius cannot deny that there will be similar effects [in both]. . . . True physicians observe the anatomy of places in the body with regard to the places of the planets . . . thus did Paracelsus speak of a double anatomy."[56]

There are, therefore, tinctures and *astra* which "contrive the dissolution of bodies and souls and which introduce the anatomy of disease into life's republic."[57] The *ens veneni* is the principle of dissolution in nature, contained as *astra* in the visible firmament and communicated to all mixed bodies in the terrestrial world. Here, especially, the text closely follows Severinus, for the *ens veneni* are seeds which, in Severinus's view, account for the return to the abyss or night of physical things. The relationship between the macrocosm and microcosm affects things in the inferior world in other ways, of course. *Astra* also communicate the vital principle from which the characteristics and qualities of all things arise. Thus "in the inferior world we see that crystal and stones are cold by nature. [But] these same properties are endowed by the visible stars. The magnet has an attractive virtue which exists also in the stars." Such operations the *Introductio* ascribes not to the heat and cold of the stars themselves but to the principles of which they consist. "Without the stars we cannot live, since heat and cold, and the arrangement of all natural things . . . arise from them."[58]

[55] *Introductio in vitalem philosophiam* (n.47), in *Opera Omnia*, 7:p. 19, cols. 1 and 2.

[56] *Introductio in vitalem philosophiam* (n.47), in *Opera Omnia*, 7:pp. 21, col 2—23, col. 1.

[57] *Introductio in vitalem philosophiam* (n.47), in *Opera Omnia*, 7:p. 18, col. 2.

[58] *Introductio in vitalem philosophiam* (n.47), in *Opera Omnia*, 7:p. 19, col. 1.

In tracing the causes of disease to *astra* as opposed to humors, the text emphasizes the importance of an astral physician like Paracelsus. Its approach to cures, however, is not exclusively through the stars. The stars indeed do their dirty work and there are, as a result, impurities mixed with everything that exists. But illnesses that arise from those impurities in the human body can be cured only with their evacuation. As we shall see Hartmann's own medical therapy and his chemical pharmacy rested largely upon the use of purgatives, including all manner of diaphoretic and sudorific preparations. In this way, he closely follows the observations of the *Introductio* that "no method can be invented which is better for curing astral illnesses and for quickly expelling the *ens veneni* than that which is by means of sweating."[59]

One of the most popular diaphoretic preparations of the early seventeenth century was *antimonium diaphoreticum*, a preparation made by burning antimony (sulphide) with saltpeter. As we will see later, Hartmann was especially fond of medicines made from antimony and recommended several sorts of antimony preparations as purgatives. The theoretical basis for those prescriptions is important to understand since it reflects something of Hartmann's deep commitment both to the astral nature of disease and to the close connection between the "inferior heaven," man, and the world at large.

In thinking about diseases and their cures Hartmann relied upon Paracelsus's model, which treated each illness as a specific entity linked to corresponding *astra* and affecting specific parts of the body. Cures, like diseases themselves, were really sorts of "transplantations" or "regenerations." In removing obstructions in the lungs occasioned by consumption (*phthisis*), for example, the physician must not only treat the blockage, in this case by prescribing spirit of vitriol, but must also restore the temperament and constitution of an "inferior heaven." Since all acute illnesses fall under the power of Saturn in the larger world, Saturn's influence in the smaller world of man must also be supplanted. The physician, in short, has to bring about a "transmutation of nature" whereby a venereal remedy replaces the saturnine illness. "If Saturn holds the keys of power in all chronic diseases, antimony holds Saturn captive

[59] *Introductio in vitalem philosophiam* (n.47), in *Opera Omnia*, 7:p. 23, col. 2.

and thus does Saturn surrender its scepter to Venus."[60] Antimony itself not only removes all obstructions "by a specific virtue," but thereafter "creates a new heaven, consuming the opposite by a fiery power . . . while renovating all of nature." These things constitute the "mysteries of cures." But it is, nevertheless, by such means that "all the *astra* in the microcosm can be transplanted and . . . human nature restored by the secrets (*arcanis*) of remedies."[61] Medicines linked to the stars thus help restore the micro-heaven of the human body. Of all the remedies that can be made, however, transplantation or regeneration results best from "those preparations involving [the combination of] antimony and other things."[62]

Paracelsus considered *phthisis* to be a tartar of the lungs, and it is to Paracelsus's tartar doctrine, detailed especially in his *De causa et origine morborum*,[63] that the *Introductio* also turns when discussing how the *ens veneni* produces illnesses of different sorts in various parts of the body. All things, although perfect in themselves, when used as food have mixed within them impurities arising from the astral presence of the *ens veneni*. Paracelsus's opinion was "that the body has been given to us without poison, and in it there is no poison. However, in that which we must give our body as nourishment there is poison. The body is created perfect, but the other is not. For that reason, when such bodies, animals and fruits, become food for us, they also are a poison. In themselves, however, they are neither poison nor food, but are, just as we are, perfect creatures." [64]

[60] *Introductio in vitalem philosophiam* (n.47), in *Opera Omnia*, 7:p. 42, col. 1.

[61] *Introductio in vitalem philosophiam* (n.47), in *Opera Omnia*, 7:p. 23, col. 1.

[62] *Introductio in vitalem philosophiam* (n.47), in *Opera Omnia*, 7:p. 23, col. 1.

[63] This is the third book of Paracelsus's *Opus paramirum*. Paracelsus's tartar doctrine is detailed in Walter Pagel, *Paracelsus: An Introduction to Philosophical Medicine in the Era of the Renaissance* (Basel and New York: S. Karger, 1958), pp. 152–165. More recently, Wolfgang Schneider (ed.), *Paracelsus—Neues von Seiner Tartarus-Vorlesung (1527/28)*, Braunschweiger Veröffentlichungen zur Geschichte der Pharmazie und der Naturwissenschaften, vol. 29 (Stuttgart: Deutscher Apotheker Verlag, 1985).

[64] Paracelsus, *Volumen Paramirum*, in *Theophrastus Paracelsus Werke: Medizinische Schriften*, ed. Will-Erich Peuchert (Basel-Stuttgart: Schwabe Verlag, 1976), vol. 1, p. 195.

When mixed in food the *ens veneni* comprises "a mucilaginous and tartarous impurity that in itself does not possess an expulsive virtue, but rather binds things together and hardens them."[65] In the human body it is the *archeus* in the stomach that separates the pure from tartarous impurities, transmuting that which is healthful into a tincture for the preservation of life. When, however, the *spagyrus* of the body does not separate correctly, there follows putrefaction and corruption, which is the mother of all illness and the source for the generation of disease. On such occasions a mucilaginous and stony substance remains and is collected into a sand, which is also called tartar.[66]

So, the *ens veneni* of the inferior world generates tartar, and following Paracelsus, the *Introductio* differentiates four tartarous types: *calculum*, *arenam*, *balum*, and *viscum*. Each is really a form of natural excrement. Just as the excrement of man is "an impure, stinking sulphur" separated by means of the stomach, there is an excrement of the natural world which is "a mucilaginous and tartarous material called by Paracelsus the salt of a thing." It is this that, unless expelled from the body, is collected into tartarous species.[67]

For the purpose of finding the *locus* of disease within specific parts of the body it is important to understand that separation and expulsion of the *ens veneni* or tartarous impurities does not occur solely in the stomach. The excrement of natural things is inherent deep in the food and drink brought into the body, and the *archeus* of the stomach alone is not able to separate it out entirely. Thus, additional separations follow, the *ens veneni* being subjected to the action of the liver, kidneys, bladder, and intestines. Indeed:

> . . . every part of the body has its peculiar stomach [*ventriculus*] that separates impurities from nutriment and gives rise to tinctures . . . . Separation in the stomach suffices [only] for nourishing the parts of the body. Thus it is necessary that there be separation in each of the body's parts so that the stomach of any of the parts separates nutriment . . . from excrement which leaves the body *via emunctoria*—the lungs through spit, the brain

[65] *Introductio in vitalem philosophiam* (n.47), in *Opera Omnia*, 7:p. 24, col. 1.

[66] *Introductio in vitalem philosophiam* (n.47), in *Opera Omnia*, 7:p. 24, col. 1.

[67] *Introductio in vitalem philosophiam* (n.47), in *Opera Omnia*, 7:p. 24, col. 2.

through the nose, the spleen through veins. . . . From this excrement tartar is generated in the principle members of the body . . . [and these are] . . . of the most subtle kind. . . . For the body of tartar is volatile and has a vaporific substance.[68]

In all parts of the body, then, there are *ventriculi* and in each special "stomach" there also is the fire of digestion and the separation of the pure from the impure. The impurities are really excrements originally of a spiritual nature owing to the presence of the *ens veneni* but assuming a subtle body following digestion and separation. For:

It is the constant decree of philosophers everywhere that the nature of bodies and spirits is reciprocal: bodies are resolved into spirits and spirits are transmuted into bodies. Therefore blood, flesh, and marrow have their own stomachs and their own digestion, separation, excrements, and tartar. The excrement of blood washes away through sweat, the excrement of flesh through urine . . . the excrement of marrow affects the dryness of the bones. The nutriments of blood, marrow, and flesh are plainly spiritual and invisible, but their excrements are visible. Nevertheless, they are the most subtle of all the parts of the body.[69]

Following Paracelsus, Hartmann believed that medicines cured disease by helping the *ventriculi* in the various parts of the body separate and then expel what had come into the body mixed with food and drink as a spiritual *ens veneni*. This was, of course, not the only source of disease, and the *Vital Philosophy* discusses other disease origins such as the *ens semenis*, the source of hereditary illnesses. But while accepting Paracelsus's descriptions of diseases arising from food, external impressions, or hereditary "seeds," the text draws the line at explanations that transcend natural causes. Thus, of the five essences of disease enumerated by Paracelsus in his *Volumen medicinae paramirum*, it incorporates only three (the *ens astrorum*, *ens naturae*, and the *ens veneni*), rejecting the other two. Paracelsus's *ens magicum* it declares to be diametrically opposed to the Christian man, while Paracelsus's *ens divinum* is occult and inaccessible to investigation [*impervestigabile*].[70]

[68] *Introductio in vitalem philosophiam* (n.47), in *Opera Omnia*, 7:p. 25, cols. 1 and 2.

[69] *Introductio in vitalem philosophiam* (n.47), in *Opera Omnia*, 7:p. 26, col. 2.

[70] *Introductio in vitalem philosophiam* (n.47), in *Opera Omnia*, 7:pp. 27, col. 1—28, col. 2.

Libavius's Response

For Libavius, making assumptions about the existence of invisible *astra* or the double anatomy of man amounted to forms of Paracelsian fantasy. Among those who had, in his opinion, most fallen victim to such fantasies and who were therefore especially responsible for having raised Paracelsus to the status of a "pseudo-monarch," were Oswald Croll, Henningus Scheunemann, Joachimn Tanckius (1557–1609), Petrus Severinus, and Johannes Hartmann. Also, the recently appearing Rosicrucian texts, the *Fama fraternitatis* (1614) and the *Confessio fraternitatis* (1615) (both published at Kassel by Wilhelm Wessel) had been, according to Libavius, inspired by Paracelsian thinking. Like them, the texts of Paracelsian authors contained gross impieties and lacked any convincing logical foundation, since each rejected altogether the value of Peripatetic philosophy.[71] Owen Hannaway has shown that for Libavius the philosophy of Aristotle was preferable to all other ancient systems of thought because it was, as he saw it, the least removed from Christian teachings. Nevertheless, in his polemics with Paracelsians, it was not so much the defense of Aristotle that concerned him as it was the condemnation of an epistemological anarchy which he considered to be implicit within Paracelsian philosophy. For Libavius, the Paracelsian reliance upon revelation, or "the light of nature," as a means of understanding relationships between the macrocosm and microcosm meant replacing an entire tradition of pious learning with the enthusiasms of personal inspiration and divine illumination.[72] This is the really dangerous part of thinking that man is a microcosm. After all, that sort of reasoning might lead to the claim that he who understands himself fundamentally knows all things. That, according to Libavius, was certainly the opinion of Cornelius Agrippa, who taught that the way to true wisdom and perpetual beatitude was to know oneself, "because the true and real nature of all things is in man."[73]

[71] Libavius, *D.O.M.A. Prodromus vitalis philosophiae Paracelsistarum de gentilium literarum autoritate, et in caussis rerum humanarum reddendis facultate* in *Appendix necessaria syntagmatis arcanorum chymicorum* . . . (1615), pp. 3–12.

[72] Hannaway, *The Chemists and the Word* (n.1), pp. 104–106.

[73] Libavius, *De philosophia vivente seu vitali Paracelsi iuxta P. Severinum . . . ex repititione I. Hartmanni* . . . in the section *Examen philosophiae novae* . . . (1615) of *Appendix necessaria syntagmatis arcanorum chymicorum* (1615), p. 253.

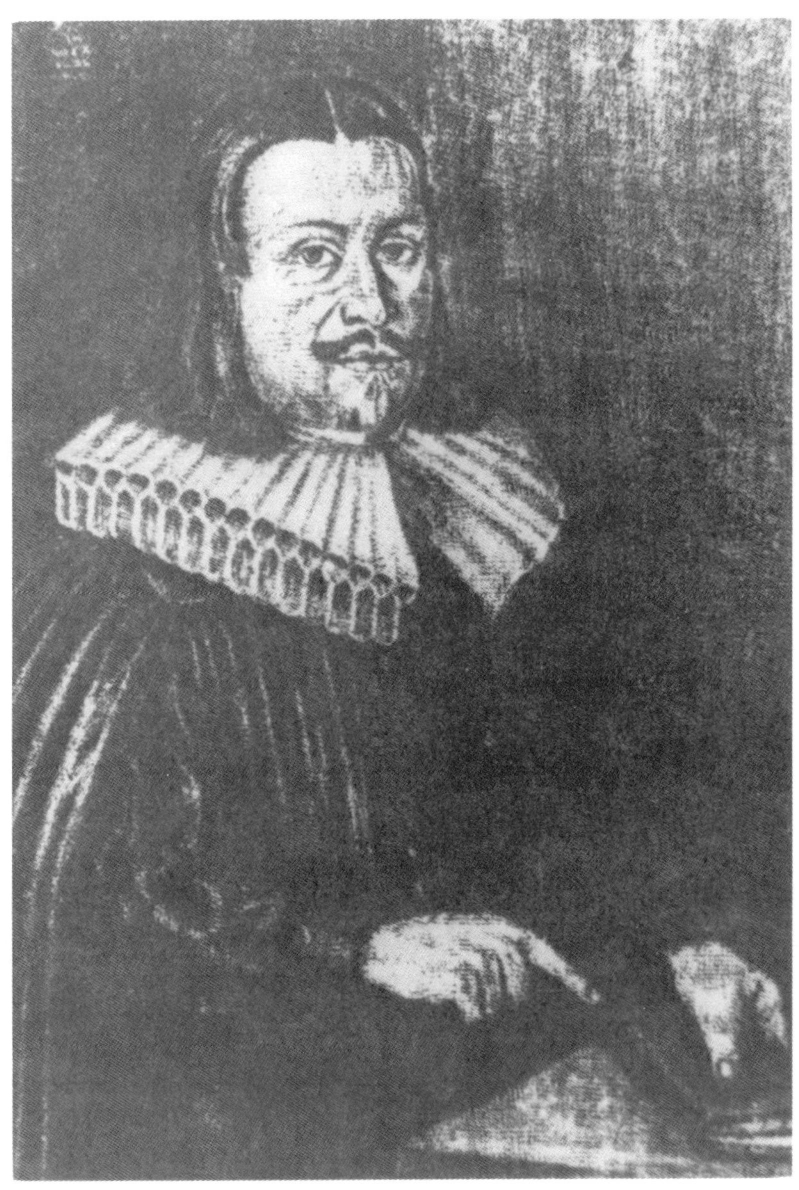

Andreas Libavius (1540–1616).

Moreover, to displace the traditional locus of intellectual authority in favor of personal experience was to deny the value of the traditional institutions of education. In the same way that religious mystics had elevated a subjective communion with God above the institutional authorities in church and state,[74] Paracelsian subjectivity, from Libavius's point of view, also involved a turning away from the historically mediated, institutionalized forms of knowledge, relying instead upon a source of learning interior to the individual.[75] Hannaway nicely sums up Libavius's fears in a quotation drawn from the first part of the *Appendix necessaria*: "Take away schoolmasters and books, and let everyone philosophize for himself without the aid of either and you will have philosophical war."[76] If Libavius read the *Introductio*, he had not far to look for the first signs of the epistemological assumptions that he felt would throw philosophy into confusion. The author had discussed academic and Peripatetic philosophy at the outset of the little treatise praising Plato, Aristotle, and others who had taught that the world had been created by God and consisted of a universal matter.[77] However, the following section, *De philosophia Hermetica et Hippocratica*, Hartmann defined philosophy as the breath of God (*spiraculum Dei*) and as divine illumination (*divina illustratio*) which lay within the power and reason of no man, but depended entirely upon divine blessing. For this reason only a few were able to acquire wisdom and truth which came as gifts from God.[78]

It is this view of philosophy that made Hartmann's position within the university at Marburg such a horror to Libavius. The seeds of philosophical evil, whose fruits denied the basis of institutional learning, had been planted within the institution itself. Paracelsians thought of the wisdom of Aristotle as an insane wisdom. But what then, Libavius asks, referring to Hartmann's incongruous position within the Marburg faculty, of

[74] See Steven Ozment, *Mysticism and Dissent: Religious Ideology and Social Protest in the Sixteenth Century* (New Haven and London: Yale University Press, 1973).

[75] Ozment, *Mysticism and Dissent* (n.74), pp. 55ff.

[76] Hannaway, *The Chemists and the Word* (n.1), p. 104.

[77] *Introductio in vitalem philosophiam* (n.47), in *Opera Omnia*, 7:pp. 1, col. 1—2, col. 1.

[78] *Introductio in vitalem philosophiam* (n.47), in *Opera Omnia*, 7:p. 2, cols. 1–2.

all those who still teach that wisdom within the Marburg academy? "Is your school really the college of insane wisdom?" "Listen to this," he instructs:

> Aristotle was a mathematician, a grammarian, and a good dialectician. He was also not a bad rhetorician. In physics he has shed such light that even your Calvinist theologians cannot do without it. Has there, therefore, been insane wisdom introduced into sacred writings? . . . Granted, Aristotle made errors in ethics, but for all that he was a better Christian and more of an enlightened philosopher than you and all like you. I don't think you have ever known anything about his philosophy. For you crept out of the discipline of mathematics and slipped straight into the Paracelsian kitchen.[79]

Libavius intended to hit hard. The slap included a physiognomic insult. Libavius added that Hartmann's abnormally shaped head (*heteroclitum caput*) was better suited for mathematics than either chemistry or medicine.[80] Knowing that Hartmann was by training a mathematician and had studied medicine and *chymiatria* only after tasting the patronage of the Kassel court, Libavius aimed straight at what he thought to be the weak philosophical underside of Hartmann's academic experience. Instead of studying Aristotle, Hartmann had stepped into the labyrinth of Egyptian wisdom. He had read about vital principles, powers, and seeds in the work of Petrus Severinus, had swallowed down *hermetica*, that is "the foolish *theologemata* of the *Pimander* and *Asclepius*," and, rather than choosing the light of Peripatetic philosophy, had preferred to ponder "dark doctrines." Such dark things had their advantage. After all, Libavius writes, it is because of the darkness that Hartmann appears great. Darkness now pervaded the Marburg lecture hall to the extent that students were forced to struggle for knowledge in the same way that a certain kind of Roman gladiator had been forced to fight blindfolded. "Oh Hartmann," Libavius exclaims, "yours is a mental darkness [*caligo*] stitched together from falsehoods, deceptions, parables, and obscure enigmas. . . . The schools of the entire world and the new and old wisdom alike are a disgrace to you because they will not be gulped down with your Paracelsian muck [*stercora tua Paracelsica*]."[81]

[79] Libavius, *De philosophia vivente* (n.73), p. 93.
[80] Libavius, *De philosophia vivente* (n.73), p. 99.
[81] Libavius, *De philosophia vivente* (n.73), pp. 93–95.

Libavius's rhetoric of darkness as applied to Hartmann's Paracelsian beliefs and to his teaching at Marburg builds upon the theme of "the night" or "Netherworld" found in the writings of the Danish Paracelsian Petrus Severinus (1542–1602), whose ideas lay at the heart of the *Vital Philosophy*. Especially Severinus's notion of "seeds" (*semina*), described as indestructible spiritual entities possessing the radical power of life, received a prominent place in the discussion. Through a process of periodic ebbing and flowing between the "abyss" or "night" and the "theater of the world," seeds brought forth and took away again all the physical bodies of nature.[82] According to Severinus, they were the spiritual links between the invisible and visible, each containing an innate knowledge of the properties of the physical bodies which it formed.[83]

Severinus too, despite his anti-Peripatetic philosophy, had attained an institutional position. Before accepting an appointment as physician to the court of the Danish king, Frederick II, he had been named *Professor paedagogicus* at the University of Copenhagen and was widely known in Paracelsian circles. His most influential work, the *Idea medicinae philosophicae* (Basel, 1571) became one of the sources most frequently cited in defense of Paracelsian doctrine at the end of the sixteenth and beginning of the seventeenth centuries. There were, to be sure, detractors. Aside from Libavius, both Thomas Erastus (1524–1583) and Daniel Sennert (1572–1637) mounted attacks against it. But the *Idea* also aroused many supporters,

[82] The notion derives from Paracelsus who viewed seeds (*semina*) as the links between material and immaterial worlds. See Walter Pagel, "Paracelsus and the Neoplatonic and Gnostic Tradition," *Ambix* 8(1960):125–166.

[83] On Severinus see Walter Pagel, *William Harvey's Biological Ideas. Selected Aspects and Historical Background* (Basel and New York: Hafner, 1967), pp. 239–247. *Idem*, *The Smiling Spleen* (Basel and New York, 1984), pp. 17–27. Allen Debus, "Petrus Severinus," *Dictionary of Scientific Biography* (New York: Scribner's, 1975), vol. 12, pp. 334–336. *Idem*, *The Chemical Philosophy: Paracelsian Science and Medicine in the Sixteenth and Seventeenth Centuries* (New York: Science History Publications, 1977), vol. I, pp. 128–131. E. Bastholm, "Petrus Severinus (1542–1602): A Danish Paracelsist," *Proceedings of the XXI International Congress of the History of Medicine* (Sienna, 1968), pp. 1080–1085. *Idem*, *Petrus Severinus og hans Idea Medicinae Philosophicae: En Dansk Paracelsist*, Acta Historica Scientiarum Naturalium et Medicinalium, vol. 32 (Odense: Odense Universitetsforlag, 1979), pp.64–73. Major advances and corrections have been brought to the study of Severinus by Jole Shackelford, "Paracelsianism in Denmark and Norway" (n.30).

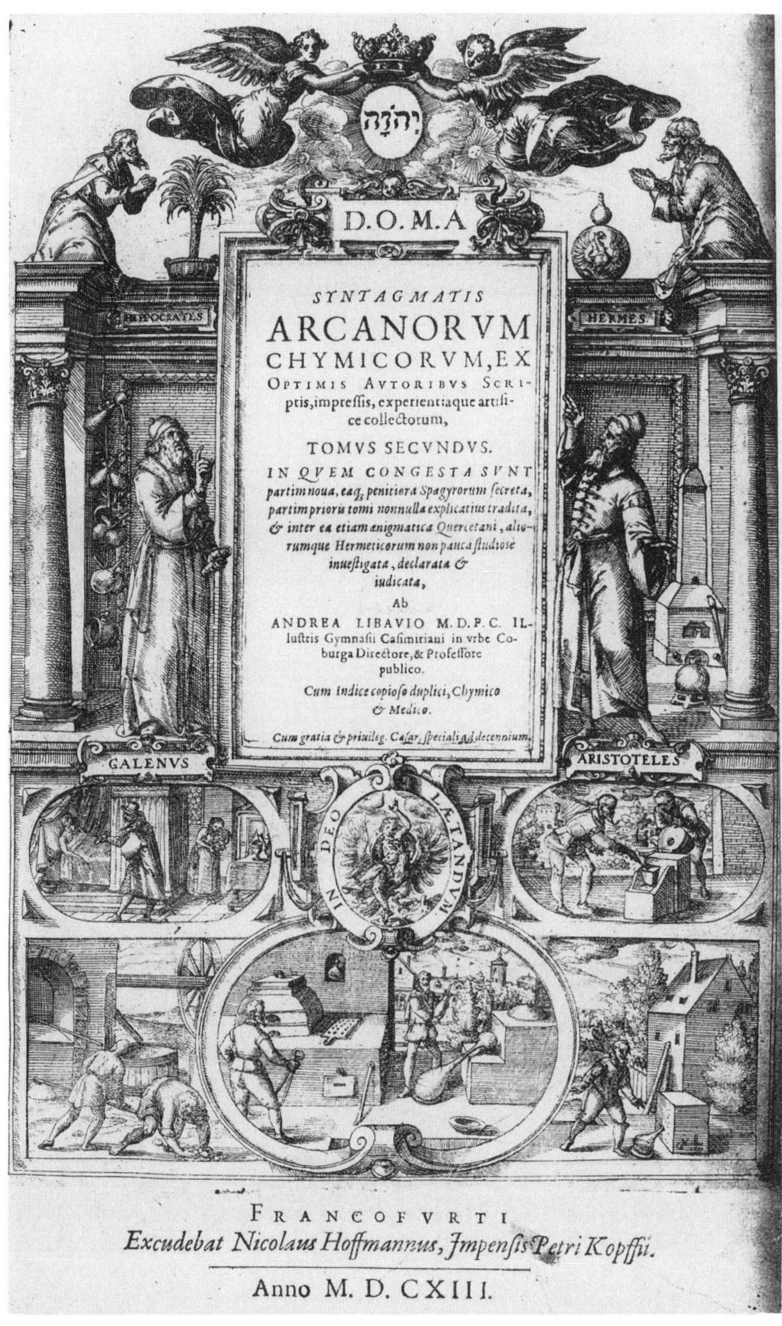

D.O.M.A

HIPPOCRATES

HERMES

SYNTAGMATIS
ARCANORVM
CHYMICORVM, EX
OPTIMIS AVTORIBVS SCRI-
ptis, impressis, experientiaque artifi-
ce collectorum,

TOMVS SECVNDVS.

IN QVEM CONGESTA SVNT
partim noua, eaq; penitiora Spagyrorum secreta,
partim prioris tomi nonnulla explicatius tradita,
& inter ea etiam ænigmatica Quercetani, alio-
rumque Hermeticorum non pauca studiosè
inuestigata, declarata &
iudicata,

Ab

ANDREA LIBAVIO M.D.P.C. IL-
lustris Gymnasii Casimiriani in vrbe Co-
burga Directore, & Professore
publico.

Cum Indice copioso duplici, Chymico
& Medico.

Cum gratia & priuileg. Cæsar. speciali ad decennium.

GALENVS

ARISTOTELES

IN DEO LÆTANDVM.

FRANCOFVRTI
Excudebat Nicolaus Hoffmannus, Impensis Petri Kopffii.

Anno M. D. CXIII.

Title page of Libavius's Syntagmatis arcanorum chymicorum *(1613).*

including Johannes Hartmann, who admired Severinus's attempt to give an academic basis to vitalist cosmology by combining Paracelsian thinking and Platonic philosophy.

In one sense, then, the "Idea" of Severinus's *Idea medicinae philosophicae* might be understood as similar to the Platonic doctrine of "forms." When combined with the philosophy of Paracelsus, however, "Idea" took on another meaning. It became a vital natural principle (*principium vitale in natura*) accounting for the life and development of all things in nature. Libavius, of course, was beyond being fooled by Paracelsian slight of hand. Joining Paracelsus to Plato was, in his view, only a thinly veiled attempt to clothe an epistemology based still on special revelation in the dress of institutionalized pedagogy. Hartmann and Severinus were guilty of the same offense—propounding Paracelsian enthusiasms in the guise of academic wisdom.

The desire to make Paracelsian philosophy seem connected to traditions possessing some degree of institutional respectability is one of the reasons why Severinus and Hartmann both argued hard to enlist Hippocrates as an ancient supporter. The Hippocratic text, *On Ancient Medicine*, had indeed been critical of humoral theory based upon qualities. Instead, Hippocrates had introduced "forces" defined as "the astringent," "the acid," "the bitter," and "the sweet." According to Severinus, Hippocrates had also relied upon a vital principle in nature, called *logoi* or *rationes*, by means of which nature, through propagation, was able to reveal itself and everything contained in it. Other points of contact led through a Hippocratic work called *De diaeta*. There the body was compared to a circle having no beginning nor end. No matter what the connection, making Hippocrates serve Paracelsian and Hermetic medicine was abhorrent to Libavius, and much of his critique of Paracelsian thinking, particularly that of Severinus and Hartmann, was aimed at distinguishing Hippocratic from hermetic medical philosophy.[84]

According to Severinus, seeds, i.e., the spiritual roots of things, emerged from "the abyss" or "night" (a state of potency) at times preordained by God to become physical bodies. Holding to the same divine time schedule, they thereafter

[84] Pagel, *William Harvey's Biological Ideas* (n.83),pp. 239–247. Also, Severinus, *Idea medicinae philosophicae* (n.83), cap. II.

passed once again back into the "night." Severinus insisted that this was not a creation from nothing, but a flux and reflux between the "night" and the physical world of the various species of existence. At appointed times, the seed that had produced a visible species simply passed once again back into the invisible netherworld. Thus, species in the physical world were constantly replenished by incorporeal bodies (seeds) viewed as emerging from the "night" and entering the mundane theater by virtue of an innate knowledge which they possessed, i.e., the "Idea" of the shape and structure of the thing to be fashioned and its predetermined time and place in the harmony of the universe. All life was really immortal, the relation between "night" and physical nature being thought of by Severinus as "cyclically returning" and "round."[85]

Along with the doctrine of seeds much of Severinus's *Idea medicinae philosophicae* concerned the elements and the principles of nature. Like Paracelsus, he considered the elements to be both spiritual and material, referring to them also as matrices or wombs in which objects were generated and from which they acquired both their signatures and specific natures. In Severinus's view, each seed was connected to a specific elemental matrix which he considered to be a spaceless and dimensionless "empty place." The elements also possessed forces, also not of the material world, which Severinus called *astra*. When combined with the chemical principles, sulphur, salt, and mercury, they connected the highest to the lowest in nature and maintained thereby a predetermined order in the universe.[86]

Everything that came into physical existence was, therefore, a spiritual mixture of an innate tincture or seed with the insensible elements and natural principles.[87] The mixture was the means by which seeds, the incorporeal elements (*astra*), and the principles of bodies achieved a synthesis and produced a new being. There needed to be an agent responsible for producing the mixture and guiding the combination of its parts, and Severinus supplied just such a dynamic principle by referring to the vital principle, the vitalistic "Idea" itself.

Since physical bodies were really composites of material and spiritual elements, seeds, and chemical principles, decompos-

[85] Severinus, *Idea medicinae philosophicae* (n.84), cap. VIII. Shackelford, "Paracelsianism in Denmark and Norway" (n.30), chapter 2.

[86] Severinus, *Idea medicinae philosophicae* (n.84), cap. V.

[87] Severinus, *Idea medicinae philosophicae* (n.84), cap. IX.

ing physical mixtures by means of fire was the best way to seek knowledge of nature. In this way, too, the practitioner also gained access to the secrets of medicine, since the seeds of each mixture could be absorbed by more powerful seeds or tinctures. Thus, says Severinus, steel is transplanted from the roots of lead, emerald from the roots of copper, and sapphire from the roots of silver.[88]

Claims of being able to prepare medicines by means of transplantation or transmutation were, for Libavius, marks of Paracelsian dishonesty, for no true chemist, in his opinion, would set out to eliminate the material matrix of things. Where the true chemist used the fire to release the interior substance of a thing, he did so without freeing its spiritual essence of all material connection.[89] Moreover, to Libavius, Severinus's natural philosophy, like the panaceas which he recommended, carried weight only as Platonic fables. Like Hermes and his followers, Severinus also had sought to lead the unsuspecting to "the back of the heavens," where Platonic ideas become separated from bodies. There one would be fooled into believing that one was contemplating nature. But, Libavius admonishes, one ought to know that nature can be contemplated only in things themselves.[90]

In giving reality to unseen *astra* which exist apart from physical bodies, Hartmann and Severinus had fallen, in Libavius's opinion, into a special sort of abyss of their own. For, he argues, if reality consists of *astra* or seeds, and this world is the mere garment [*indumentum*] of another, what should one believe about the resurrection of the dead? Certainly Hartmann must know that if he dies in the Lord, and not in Calvin, he will see the Lord in his own flesh. But, "if this world is ghostly and the scene of fables . . . who shall see God?" In the philosophy of Paracelsus it is the sidereal and spiritual man that is fit for immortality, while the elementary body is discarded as the dross of nature.[91] Actually, for Hartmann, the real God is not the Christian God at all. He believes in a natural God, the origin of all

[88] Severinus, *Idea medicinae philosophicae* (n.84). According to Severinus, species may be wholly changed when their elements and principles receive different signatures. See Shackelford, "Paracelsianism in Denmark and Norway" (n.30), pp. 99–102.

[89] Hannaway, *The Chemists and the Word* (n.1), pp. 87–88.

[90] Libavius, *De philosophia vivente* (n.73), p. 128.

[91] Libavius, *De philosophia vivente* (n.73), p. 162.

things, called Mercury.[92] There is, Libavius concludes, nothing pious in this philosophy, and he advises Hartmann "to take the hellebore," (a plant considered a remedy for madness) before the philosophy of Paracelsus drives him totally insane.[93]

On Libavius's account the similarities between Platonic and Hermetic reasoning are nowhere more obvious than in the way Paracelsians like Hartmann treat the elements. While admitting that the world was created from four elements—earth, air, fire, and water—Hermes asserted that these were originally formed from a *materia* having the potentiality of creation but not yet created (*creabilis quidem, sed non creata*). Hermes had referred to "hyle" as the receptacle of all things in nature. Hartmann and other Paracelsians likewise imagined that out of a dark chaos there emerged a *materia prima*, a crude mass, that they called the mother of all things and the origin of all action. It was the font of life, the origin of mixtures and tinctures, and the source of the elements.[94] The Hermeticists believe this even though it is impossible, Libavius thinks, that the *prima materia* could possess all this power, for nature and soul must always be considered separate agents.[95] Paracelsians insist that the true elements are eternal and invisible and include in themselves the seeds or roots of things, which are said to produce visible fruits. However, if the elements are eternal, Libavius argues, their seeds must also be eternal, for they, like the elements, are ideas of the divine mind and exist before all things.[96]

Libavius is even more critical of Hartmann's specific notion of the elements. Not only does Hartmann subscribe to Severinus's belief in primary elements that arise in empty places and in which seeds "arise in the abyss and netherworld of Orpheus" (*nascentium in abysso et Orphei orco*), but Hartmann goes further, Libavius claims, holding ultimately to only two elements, water and earth, while insisting that air and fire possess a spiritual status only. At the same time, this *Hermes Hartmanni* distinguishes between three different sorts of elements. The first kind is pure emptiness (the divine idea). The second sort refers to material principles and are, as Croll and other Paracelsians

[92] Libavius, *De philosophia vivente* (n.73), pp. 204–205; 207–212.
[93] Libavius, *De philosophia vivente* (n.73), p. 130.
[94] Libavius, *De philosophia vivente* (n.73), pp. 181–184.
[95] Libavius, *De philosophia vivente* (n.73), p. 148.
[96] Libavius, *De philosophia vivente* (n.73), pp. 133–138.

also maintain, invisible and spiritual. The third sort comprise the external elements, the "filthy tunics" of the *astra*, seeds, balsams, tinctures, and principles of nature. But how, Libavius wonders, does something come from nothing? How do even spiritual elements arise when all that precedes them is a night and Netherworld (*nox et Orcus*) which are themselves defined as the privation of essence and the seat of darkness? If the elements and seeds are set into motion by a *prima materia* in this netherworld how can that *prima materia* be the origin of all action when it is considered to be the closest thing to Aristotelian emptiness and privation (*vacuitati et privationi Aristotelicae proximi*)? There should, Libavius advises, be a new place for the elements, seeds, and *astra* of Hartmann and Severinus, a place which is not below and not in the heavens, something, he suggests, like a papist Purgatory. In supporting this sort of Paracelsian cosmology "Hartmann," Libavius writes, "who is a stranger in physics, wanders without method."[97]

Nor is he able to be guided by Hippocrates, as he claims. For, while the fire of Hippocrates produces seeds and, when joined with water, the species of animals, this must not be confused with the hermetic fire. The seeds of Hermes emerge from the darkness [*ex orco*] and are resolved into the same. There is nothing like this in Hippocrates. Neither is there a crude mass [*rudem massam*] preceding creation in Hippocrates as there is in Hermes. Moreover what Hartmann calls *leo viridis*, the invisible principle of nature possessing the power (*potentia*) of germination, is also nowhere to be found in Hippocrates.[98]

For all these reasons, Hartmann, in Libavius's view, ought to be regarded as *Hermes Marburgicus* and *Hermes Hartmannicus*. He, like Severinus and other Paracelsians, teaches that nothing perishes, but that all things retire into the abyss. For, Hartmann thinks, if things would not return to the netherworld from which they came, new things would not be able to be born in turn, and nature would long since have been exhausted. But such a belief, Libavius contends, denies the power of divine providence and trusts instead upon the words of Hermes in the *Pimander* who says that nothing dies away in the world, there being only a dissolution of mixtures.[99]

[97] Libavius, *De philosophia vivente* (n.73), pp. 155–181.
[98] Libavius, *De philosophia vivente* (n.73), pp. 121–129.
[99] Libavius, *De philosophia vivente* (n.73), pp. 121; 189–203.

Thus, while wrapping himself in darkness, and telling fables about empty elements, Hartmann laughs at others and so distinguishes his "Sparta" (as opposed to an "Athens" presumably) in the Hessian university. He professes the philosophy of Hermes and Paracelsus, calling Peripatetic philosophers and professors of Galenic medicine "the vulgar men of the schools."[100] One would, Libavius facetiously observes, certainly never want to accept the opinions of anyone who had earned the reputation of being an "ass of the schools" (*asinus de Schola*). "Although," he adds, "there is one who lives in the school of Marburg."[101] Indeed, holding forth in the Marburg lecture hall is a person who, in place of a most pure and chaste philosophy, rejoices "in the dung of hogs and in belchings from the drunkenness of Paracelsus."[102] It is not the love of philosophy that moves this man but the love of making money through the sale of purgatives. "Paracelsians gulp down panaceas made hastily for all persons, illnesses, affectations, and times. You [Hartmann] sell your vomitory (*Speywasser*) in great amounts. But for what reason? With your leave I will tell you: solely for the sake of *Auripeta*[103] . . . And thus do you embrace the land of Hesse so sweetly that your store of money swells, or do the Hessians disgorge themselves only of soul (*animam*)?"[104]

Evidently, Hartmann's spiritual philosophy did not prevent him from having something physical to sell. Neither did that philosophy interfere with teaching the preparation of chemical medicaments in the Marburg laboratory. As we will see, Hartmann cashed in here as well. Students promised an honorarium to their instructor, not for philosophical disclosures, but for practical information and guidance in the making of medicines. What those medicines were and how students went about preparing them will be the focus of the section to follow.

[100] Libavius, *De philosophia vivente* (n.73), pp. 100; 161.
[101] Libavius, *De philosophia vivente* (n.73), p. 100.
[102] Libavius, *De philosophia vivente* (n.73), p. 246.
[103] That is, tinfoil gilded with a linseed oil glaze. See Edmund O. von Lippmann, *Entstehung und Ausbreitung der Alchemie* (Berlin: Springer, 1919), I: pp. 466, 473.
[104] Libavius, *De philosophia vivente* (n.73), p. 249.

PART TWO

The Practical Component of Academic *Chymiatria*

The Rules of the Laboratory and the Duties of Teacher and Student

Hartmann referred to the university place reserved for pharmaceutical instruction under his guidance as a public chemico-medical laboratory. While the term *laboratorium* is used, we should not immediately think that it had much in common with modern counterparts. From references in the diary we can piece together that Hartmann's *laboratorium* was furnished with glass and earthen vessels including bowls and containers of various types and was equipped with the typical sorts of distillation apparatus, primarily retorts and alembics. There were also water and sand baths for the slow distillation or digestion of substances, and ovens, a knowledge of whose construction students were expected to acquire as part of their laboratory experience. Various tools including spatulas, tongs, and a balance came into play in the course of progressing through operations recorded by Hartmann. As we shall see, students also had access to a variety of chemical substances stored in the laboratory, most of which probably had been purchased at the Frankfurt fair. There were also servants in the laboratory helping in the elementary preparations, cleaning up, and, most importantly, tending to the fires when Hartmann and his students were away.

In contrast to many alchemical work spaces, Hartmann's *laboratorium* was a fixed space and we know quite a lot about the projects undertaken in that space due to a laboratory notebook kept for two semesters beginning in the same year that Libavius published his *Appendix necessaria syntagmatis*,

1615.[1] As we shall see, the diary was both a notebook, recording procedures in the laboratory on a day to day basis, and an informal textbook. However, access to the textbook was limited to Hartmann's own students.

In his introduction, Hartmann welcomes students to the study of the art of Apollo in the place sacred to Apollo and Hermes.[2] Gaining access to that place required students to agree to specific responsibilities and to a prescribed relationship to their teacher. Their first obligation was to pray everyday for the well-being and longevity (*pro incolumitate ac longaevitate*) of prince Moritz, the Landgrave of Hesse, the renowned founder and patron of chemical studies within the university. Just as important, however, was their loyalty to the director of their college and Hartmann made the first of twenty-one introductory points the requirement that all students take an oath (*sacramentum dicere*), swearing to him their obedience, faithfulness, diligence, discretion, and gratitude before stepping foot into the laboratory itself. Along with any rebellious frame of mind they were also to leave all forms of baggage, including coats and swords, at the laboratory entrance. Since students would be personally involved in the preparation of medicaments, they were also to see to the protection of their clothes by providing themselves with a little skirt (*castula*) or a linen apron. At this point, properly attired for the work ahead, committed to observing perfect courtesy and obedience to their teacher, and dutifully grateful for the benefi-

[1] A copy of Hartmann's record of laboratory procedures (MS 1207) and other Hartmann autographs make up parts of the manuscript collection of the *Universitätsbibliothek* in Erlangen. Hans Fischer, *Katalog der Handschriften der Universitätsbibliothek Erlangen* (*Die Lateinischen Papierhandschriften*) (Erlangen: Universitätsbibliothek, 1936), vol. 2. Although a brief review of the document and a partial transcription appeared in 1941, the author, W. Ganzenmüller, focused only upon procedures concerning the making of *laudanum* and *laudanum opiatum* in the first of the two courses represented in the diary. Accompanying procedures from the first course, and those making up the whole of the second, were not described. See W. Ganzenmüller, "Das chemische Laboratorium der Universität Marburg im Jahre 1615," *Angewandte Chemie* 54(1941): 215–217. While Ganzenmüller's treatment can be regarded as, for the most part, precise. Some inaccuracies, especially regarding the names and numbers of students enrolled in Hartmann's courses, also exist. These I have tried to correct in the following account.

[2] A record of Hartmann's opening instructions to students comprise Universitätsbibliothek Erlangen: MS 1207, pp. V-VIII. (Hereafter Erlangen). Ganzenmüller, "Das chemische Laboratorium" (n.1), pp. 215–216.

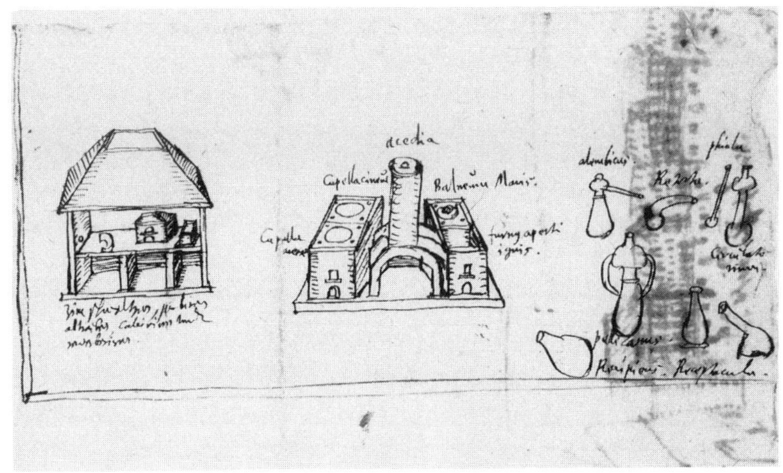

Drawings of the Landgrave Moritz of Hessen of alchemical-pharmaceutical apparatus, from Murhardsche Bibliothek, Kassel 2° Ms Hass. 107.

cence of the university's patron, students entered a place reserved for the communication of a special, indeed privileged, form of knowledge.

Once inside that space the focus of Hartmann's instructions to students takes an interesting turn aimed at insuring correct behavior in regard to the new physical environment. Students are encouraged to look at everything and to ask about the processes underway, but to do so with modesty and without becoming an annoyance. They should be neither idle nor negligent when in the laboratory, and should always listen carefully to what is being taught and demonstrated. No one will be allowed to take away anything from the laboratory without the director's knowledge. Neither should students extort anything by force or by deceit from the servants. The types of chemical utensils and especially the construction of the ovens were to be carefully observed. Indeed, students ought to be able to construct ovens for themselves. In their notes, they should record the ingredients of preparations and should carefully set down the degrees and times of the fire. Care must also be taken not to break any of the chemical instruments. If there is damage, however, the person responsible must bear the cost of replacement.

Working through preparations was serious business and Hartmann was not keen on interruptions. Students were to avoid clattering about and were given strict warnings against yelling, drinking, sleeping, and fighting. Each was expected to look after his own notebook, to take part in the day-to-day work in the laboratory, and to arrive punctually except when delayed by necessity or as a result of attending public lectures. Either as a way to instill a sense of community among students or to lessen the demand for personal attention, Hartmann encouraged his students to help one another in the laboratory. They were, however, never to handle anything without his consent. After removing chemicals for the purpose of exploring their nature and uses, they must also make sure to put them back again carefully.

The final points of Hartmann's *laboratorii publici chymico-medici in illustri academia Marburgensi leges* ("rules of the public chemico-medical laboratory in the illustrious Marburg academy") mostly concern the need for secrecy about the work to be undertaken. Although a public laboratory, it is clear that Hartmann considered the knowledge imparted there to be privileged and thought of his students as taking part in something like a secret society. What they have seen, heard, experienced or otherwise come into possession of as result of their work, he instructs, may not be divulged to the unworthy nor be made public, for such would amount to deceiving their teacher and be a violation of divine law. Rather, students should serve one another, and not abuse the director's kindness. After leaving the laboratory, their public and private lives should testify to their gratitude. In concluding remarks, Hartmann tells his students to extol these noble studies (i.e., the preparations of chemical medicines) everywhere and to advance them in their own work to the best of their abilities. All this should be done in the name of the most holy Jehovah. Anyone acting otherwise or seriously failing in his duties, Hartmann warns, shall be excluded from the college and shut out of the fellowship.

Only at this point does Hartmann's laboratory notebook really begin. The content of the first semester's instruction is clear from the title: "Diary of the daily chemical operations in the preparation of opium and *laudanum opiatum*, as well as the preparation of English Potable Gold, and of other useful chemicals, in the months July and August and until the autumn fair, 1615." Before demonstrations began, however, there was one matter yet to be considered: how the instructor would be paid and what he would promise in return. In other words, students and teacher needed to sign a contract. As it turns out, that contract tells us much about mutual obligations in the laboratory and is especially relevant to understanding what Hartmann perceived as his role in fashioning a laboratory didactic.

In the contract, medical students agree to participate with Dr. Johann Hartmann, public professor of *chymiatria*, in the public laboratory for the purpose of learning the preparation of opium, *laudanum opiatum*, and the ingredients of the same. They also agree to participate in the preparation of other chemical substances, especially the English Potable Gold. Hartmann promises that he will demonstrate (*monstrabit*) the preparation of opium and *laudanum opiatum* and will teach (*docebit*) the elaboration of the individual ingredients involved. Furthermore, he will explain (*explicabit*) chemical terms and phrases, "and those things that by chance will not seem clear and open enough he will render again by a clear, full, and complete setting forth of the facts" (*et quae forsan non satis clara apertaque visa fuerint, plena integraque expositione clara reddet*). He will then work out (*elaborabit*) preparations from opium and laudanum, as well as other useful things, and will faithfully demonstrate the individual procedures and necessary steps in making the *aurum potabile Angelicanum* of Francis Anthony (1550–1623), in which he will carefully train (*exercebit*) his students.[3]

Hartmann's choice of words is important. The emphasis is upon clarity in terms of both word and deed. The didactic of the laboratory is to include explanation and precise exposition but is really based upon demonstration, careful elaboration, and hands on training. This is significant both from the point of view of didactic and for what it tells us about the style of polemic Hartmann chose in confronting his primary critic, Libavius. Hartmann intended to use the laboratory as a polemical space where he could respond to Libavius not just with words, but by showing students through *praxis* the advantage of his own medical philosophy. Knowledge in the laboratory would be communicated both by what was heard and by what was observed. Students needed to listen, but much more they needed to keep their eyes open and to imitate what they saw.

And yet, all this is to take place within the context of a private conversation (*privatim dictans*) so that the meaning of "public" in Hartmann's "public chemico-medical laboratory" really ends up referring to information shared with a privileged few. In fact, on their side of the contract, students promised that they would keep silent about what was demonstrated to them. While in Marburg, as well as after their departure, they agreed not to divulge what they had learned in any sort of public writing. The relevance of "public spaces" to the production of experimental knowledge has been amply demonstrated in the writings of Steven Shapin and Simon Schaffer.[4] Hartmann's "public" *laboratorium* was public only in the sense that it was open to all interested students. Crossing its threshold, however, meant that those same students accepted the conditions of a closed, even secretive, society

[3] Erlangen (n.2), pp. VIII-X.

[4] Steven Shapin and Simon Schaffer, *Leviathan and the Air-Pump: Hobbes, Boyle, and the Experimental Life* (Princeton: Princeton University Press, 1985); Steven Shapin, "The House of Experiment in Seventeenth-Century England," *Isis* 79(1988):373–404.

bound by strict obedience to their teacher. Nevertheless, there was still a difference between Hartmann's officially public, yet personally private, *laboratorium* and other secretive spaces. The secrets that Hartmann was concerned to protect were not secrets in the mystical sense. These were rather trade secrets[5]—secrets that were knowable not through divine inspiration but by means of correct procedural instruction. In learning them, students promised to go about their work diligently and also to participate in the necessary night watches. Hartmann, for his part, agreed to pay for the ingredients in making opium and *laudanum opiatum*, but his students promised to pay him an honorarium, each according to his means, in gratitude for his teaching.[6]

Opium and Laudanum Opiatum

Signing the laboratory contract, the names of thirteen students appear with Hartmann's own. Those joining him in the laboratory made up an international group, coming from Denmark, Prussia, Poland, Silesia, as well as from neighboring German principalities.[7] One, Johann Philipp Molther, would succeed his teacher as professor of medicine and pharmacy at Marburg upon Hartmann's departure from the university in 1621 to become *Leibarzt* (personal physician to the prince) at the Kassel court.[8]

The potential appeal of *chymiatria* to an international student body had been one of the considerations that had moved Moritz of Hesse to authorize the new discipline. The university at Marburg was, like most German universities in the seven-

[5] On the tradition of "secrets" understood as recipes or "experiments," see William Eamon, "Arcana Disclosed: The Advent of Printing, the Books of Secrets, and the Development of Experimental Science in the Sixteenth Century," *History of Science* 22(1984):111–150; also, "Books of Secrets in Medieval and Early Modern Science," *Sudhoffs Archiv* 69(1985):26–49.

[6] Erlangen (n.2), pp. VIII-X. Ganzenmüller, "Das chemische Laboratorium" (n.1).

[7] These were M. Hildebrandus Küen, Nicolaus Fossius and Johann Rhodius (both from Denmark), Michael Volckman and M. Petrus Titius from Silesia, Johann Philipp Moltherus, Daniel Beckerus, Andreas Lipius from Berlin, Paulus Pauli Cleophae and Johann Stellius from Prussia, Ernst Nizenius, Simon Batkovius Losenas from Poland, and Johann Petrus Lotichius from the Wetterau.

[8] Dietrich Christoph von Rommel, *Geschichte von Hessen*, 8 vols. (Cassel, 1820–43), 6: p. 493.

teenth century, a small institution. Marburg, however, had special problems. A visitation ordered by the prince to his university in 1607 had not found the academy well attended.[9] The decline in student numbers was at least partly due to the fact that the curriculum at Marburg had grown thin owing to defections from the faculty in reaction to Moritz's own religious reforms. The Hessian prince had demanded conformity to certain so-called "points of improvement," which emphasized a particular understanding of the person of Christ and the Eucharist.[10] To some, however, the "points of improvement" appeared to be an insistence upon Calvinist doctrine. Instead of yielding to reformed religious ideas, many professors left Marburg for positions at more orthodox Lutheran universities. The medical faculty was especially hard hit. At one point students had threatened withdrawal from the university because no one could be found to lecture. By 1615, things had begun to settle down once again and the new discipline of *chymiatria* had begun to win back some of the attention to the university that had earlier been lost. For Hartmann and his thirteen students, work in the laboratory began on 10 July with the preparation of opium for the production of *laudanum opiatum*.

Laudanum had, of course, been around for a long time before Hartmann began treating it as part of his laboratory course in *chymiatria*. There was, however, considerable variation in the use of the term in ancient literature and in Paracelsus's writings. Thanks primarily to work done by Henry Sigerist in the early 1940s we know that "laudanum" was the medieval form for "ladanum" or "ledanum" which had been used before Paracelsus to refer to secretions from the leaves and flowers of different types of cistus.[11] Both Dioscorides and Galen described it and Mattioli, in his *Commentaries on Dioscorides*, gave over an entire chapter to its description and uses.

In a number of recipes Paracelsus made use of what was called *laudanum purum* which Sigerist believed to have been

[9] Heinrich Hermelink and Siegfried A. Kaehler, *Die Philipps-Universität zu Marburg, 1527–1927* (Marburg: N.G. Elwert, 1927), p. 218.

[10] Heinrich Heppe, *Die Einführung der Verbesserungspünkte in Hessen vom 1604–1610* . . . (Cassel: J.C. Krieger, 1849). Wilhelm Mauer, *Bekenntnisstand und Bekenntnis-entwicklung in Hessen* (Gütersloh: Bertelsmann, 1965).

[11] Henry E. Sigerist, "Laudanum in the Works of Paracelsus," *Bulletin of the History of Medicine* 9(1941): 530–544.

ladanum from which impurities had been removed, probably by distillation. This also could be referred to as *liquor laudani* or as *extractum laudani*. In some recipes, Paracelsus prescribed ladanum as *laudanum praeparatum* which Sigerist considered to be, at least for Paracelsus, the same as *laudanum purum*. Later Paracelsians had a different interpretation, however. For them, particularly as it appears in the work of Leonard Thurneysser and Michael Toxites, *laudanum praeparatum* was a compound remedy containing ambergris and mace.

A problem arises when Paracelsus, who on the one hand refers to laudanum in the traditional, ancient sense as a gum like mastic and myrrh, refers also to laudanum as a special sort of remedy, an arcanum, which is superior to all other medicines in instances of impending death. In this case, what Paracelsus means is a drug containing gold, pearls, and antimony. What it conspicuously does not contain, however, is opium. In this instance, and in others recounted by Sigerist, Paracelsus used laudanum as a term describing a remedy, one of many in the Paracelsian pharmacopoeia, made from pearls. He sometimes called it *laudanum perlatum*; but, whatever its name, the point is that although Paracelsus made many remedies from opium, he never discussed laudanum among them.[12]

It was then following Paracelsus, that a group of iatrochemists, a group to which Johannes Hartmann also belongs, began discussing laudanum as an opium preparation. Oswald Croll listed in his *Basilica chymica* two laudanum preparations where opium was the chief ingredient. These he called *laudanum Paracelsi laudatissimum* and *electuarium laudani*.[13] Hartmann went further. In commenting on Croll's recipes, he noted that there were numerous laudanum preparations each touted as representing Paracelsus's recipes. One of the preparations described by Croll and attributed to Paracelsus contained, besides opium, juice of henbane, which Hartmann thought unnecessary. Yet, says Hartmann, the basis of Paracelsus's composition was always opium, although another of Paracelsus's preparations, sometimes called laudanum, used gold

[12] Sigerist, "Laudanum" (n.11).

[13] Oswald Croll, *Basilica chymica continens philosophicam propria laborum experientia confirmatam descriptionem et usum remediorum chymicorum selectissimorum e lumine gratiae et naturae desumptorum* . . . (Frankfurt: G. Tampachii, 1609), pp. 173–180.

as its basic ingredient.[14] In his *Praxis chymiatrica*, a work completed by 1619[15] but published only posthumously by Johann Michaelis and Hartmann's son Georg Eberhard in 1633,[16] Hartmann collected a variety of laudanum recipes, some using opium, which, in like manner, he attributed to Paracelsus.

What procedures did Hartmann recommend, then, to his students? To prepare opium for making *laudanum opiatum* those present in the Marburg laboratory were first given an overview of the work that lay ahead. Hartmann explained that they would first take a pound of the best opium, cut it into pieces, and place the pieces into one or more bowls. The bowls would then be set on sand in a digesting oven until a "stinking sulphur" was gradually vaporized away. When the opium in the oven had given off its sulphur smell and could be ground between the fingers, Hartmann would then have his students grind the opium in a mortar, mix it with distilled vinegar, and thereafter "extract" (i.e., distill) the solution over a slow fire. The distillate would then be allowed to run through a paper, coagulated, and to each ounce would be joined a half ounce of magisteries of coral and pearl (which would also have to be prepared). To the mixture must then be added two drams of extract of crocus (another ingredient that students would need to prepare separately) and the resulting mass, thereafter, formed into pills.[17]

It is easy to know how Hartmann accounted for the effects of opium around the time he was instructing students in its preparation since, in 1615, he held a public lecture concerning opium's properties, characteristics, and medical applications. The lecture was not published, however, until after Hartmann's death, appearing at Wittenberg in 1635 as the *Tractatus physico-medicus de opio . . .*, edited by Johann

[14] *Oswaldi Crollii Basilica Chymica, pluribus selectis et secretissimis propria manuali experientia approbatis descriptionibus, et usu remediorum chymicorum selectissimorum aucta a Johanne Hartmanno* . . . in Hartmann, *Opera Omnia*, 2: p. 84, col. 2.

[15] A manuscript copy, 1619, became part of the chemical library of Moritz of Hesse. MBK: 8° MS Chem 26.

[16] I have used this edition which appears as *Johannis Hartmanni, Medicinae Doctoris et quondam chymiatriae in Academia Marburgensi professoris celeberrimi, principumque Hassiae Archiatri Praxis Chymiatrica* . . . ,in Hartmann's *Opera Omnia*, vol. 1. A second edition appeared in 1659, edited by Cardilucius.

[17] Erlangen (n.2), p. 1.

Georg Pelshofer.[18] In the treatise Hartmann discussed the etymology of opium, its place of origin, its substance and qualities, manner of collection, and the best means of distinguishing false from genuine opium before turning to its preparation and uses as a medicament.

Opium, like all worldly things, he describes as a mixed body made up from parts of the general categories of vegetables, animals, minerals, and metals.[19] It is, therefore, a separable thing and can be resolved into its individual parts by *spagyrica*, which also removes the impurities planted in it by nature. But, Hartmann insists, it is not from the traditional qualities (hot, cold, wet, and dry) that opium's narcotic effects arise. These emerge from the same general source that accounts for the action of each thing in the world. A body's efficient causes are due, he argues, to the composition of its essential principles, sulphur, salt, and mercury, which are placed by nature in the seeds of bodies, as if in the very substance of a body.[20]

To explain opium's stupefying effects Hartmann points to the agency of an oily sulphur. Yet the sulphur in opium also had a soothing and somniferous effect. "We say, therefore, that in opium, as in many other things, may indeed be seen two or more distinct actions to which a diversity of effects ought to be ascribed."[21] Thus, Hartmann advises that the "tears" (juice) of opium should be collected from a mature poppy since the sulphur within it will also be mature and make the best medicine. Some parts of all bodies, including opium, are harmful, a condition that Hartmann related to the first sin of Adam and Eve. But, by gently heating opium, the sulphurous malignity could be removed leaving behind its soothing effects and making a most wholesome anodyne. "Thus opium looses its stupefying part, but retains the soothing, sleep inducing essence."[22]

The method of heating opium to separate purities from impurities was also the procedure praised by Joseph Duchesne in a chapter entitled "de narcoticis" of his *Pharmacopoeia*

[18] *Tractatus physico-medicus de opio, a claro Viro Joh. Hartmanno . . . publice praelectus Marburgi anno 1615, nunc vero primum in lucem editus a Johannes-Georgio Pelshofero, Medic. D. et in Academia Wittenbergensi professore* (Wittenberg, 1635). In Hartmann, *Opera Omnia*, 5: pp. 2–24.

[19] *Tractatus de opio* (n.18), in *Opera Omnia*, 5:p. 12, cols. 1–2.

[20] *Tractatus de opio* (n.18), in *Opera Omnia*, 5:p. 10, col. 2-p. 18, col. 1.

[21] *Tractatus de opio* (n.18), in *Opera Omnia*, 5:p. 12, col. 2.

[22] *Tractatus de opio* (n.18), in *Opera Omnia*, 5:p. 13, col. 1.

. . . *restituta* (1607).[23] The same method, however, had been attacked by Andreas Libavius in the *Syntagmatis* (vol. 1, chap. 11), where Libavius complained that the drying up of opium destroyed the most important part of its essence. Like Hartmann, Croll, and others, Libavius believed that the noxious part of opium had to be removed before opium could be made into a useful medicine, but he did not, Hartmann recounts, "recognize this flammable, fetid sulphur as the essence of the thing." More important, from Hartmann's point of view, Libavius had misunderstood the procedure he had criticized. Rather than actually burning the opium to ashes, Hartmann and others had simply warmed the opium by a gentle fire, repeating the process many times "so that, little by little, the fetid sulphur is evaporated and emits a sweet odor and so that a dry carcass is left behind since reason and experience repeatedly testify that through the act of extraction healthful medicines are made."[24]

By contrast, Libavius recommended first dissolving opium in *aceto caryophyllato* or in *spiritu aceti*; then filtering the solution. This then (dissolving and filtering) would be repeated until the solution was pure. The pure solution needed then to be circulated in a pelican and the final pure opium liquor thereafter collected through distillation. The methods advocated by Hartmann and Libavius really hinged on whether or not fire should be used in unlocking opium's medicinal effects. Hartmann recommended the use of heat, Libavius did not. There was nothing new in that debate. In fact, the disagreement follows from one of the most common sorts of argument in alchemical literature—so common, in fact, that processes requiring the use of fire and those that did not had become generally known as "the hot way" and "the wet way" respectively.

But there was more. In Libavius's procedure, Hartmann notes that the dissolution of opium in the *acetum* causes a froth to form on the top of the solution which Libavius takes away with a spoon. Libavius believed (according to Hartmann) that the stupefying part of the opium was to be found in the froth and by removing it he would also remove opium's malignity.

[23] *D.O.M.A. Pharmacopoea Dogmaticorum Restituta pretiosis selectisque Hermeticorum floribus abunda illustrata* . . . (Paris: Claudium Morellum via Jacobaea ad signe Fontis, 1607), Chapter 24.

[24] *Tractatus de opio* (n.18), in *Opera Omnia*, 5:p. 13, col. 1.

"But," Hartmann cautions, "in the true dissolution of opium no froth, even if dissolved for the longest time, will be found."[25] In other words, even if one follows the procedure carefully, what Libavius says will happen is not borne out by laboratory experience. Libavius simply lacks sophistication in the manual operations of the laboratory and, as in a thousand chemical and alchemical debates preceding this one, experience and reason are found to reside entirely on one side. "Truly," says Hartmann, "to conjecture in chemistry is to introduce the power of experience, by which alone reason (*ratio*) is able to establish the correct method of operation."[26] Clearly, Hartmann believes that, at least in this instance, he has the greater experience and that reason will bear out his processes as he is able to demonstrate them in the laboratory before his students. The problem between Hartmann and Libavius was, therefore, not entirely a philosophical one. The two also had procedural quarrels. In fact for Hartmann, who does not talk philosophy at all when criticizing Libavius, these were the most important differences between them. It was not only, then, that his position at Marburg allowed Hartmann to advocate a spiritual view of nature as a formal part of the university curriculum that may have been repugnant to Libavius, but that Hartmann could use that position to train students to follow his own laboratory procedures while discrediting Libavius's claim to chemical experience.

Laboratory Didactic and the Production of *Laudanum Opiatum*

As we have already seen, students knew ahead of time what the general procedure was in making *laudanum opiatum*. But how did those students actually proceed from one day to the next in their laboratory work? Hartmann's laboratory diary offers us a wonderful opportunity to follow students in daily operations. In paying attention to it we are ourselves instructed, not in what could be taught, but in what actually was taught. Hartmann's diary brings an immediacy to the laboratory and to the didactic treatment of *chymiatria* that, for the most part, is unmatched by other sources in the history of early

[25] *Tractatus de opio* (n.18), in *Opera Omnia*, 5:p. 13, col. 2.
[26] *Tractatus de opio* (n.18), in *Opera Omnia*, 5:p. 13, col. 2.

modern chemistry and pharmacy. Its contents deserve a detailed survey, even though a complete understanding of student involvement in the processes described cannot be reconstructed from the remaining record. Especially, satisfactory answers to the question of which tasks fell to which students and to whether students made their own preparations or worked always in common are not forthcoming from a reading of the diary itself. For this reason, we must first get a feeling for the actual arrangement of Hartmann's laboratory notebook and for the types of entries included in it before beginning a discussion of the daily activities recorded there.

As previously mentioned, the diary recounts procedures during two academic periods corresponding to the Marburg summer and winter terms, 1615 and 1616. The focus is different for each academic quarter with the preparation of opium and the making of *laudanum opiatum* promised only for the first. Many entries refer only to individual parts of much more elaborate procedures that unfold over a series of days. With only one exception (the making of the English *aurum potabile*) the notes, which appear for each day excluding Christmas and most Sundays, are entirely impersonal. Only ingredients and laboratory procedures are listed and these are not always fully described. For that reason it will be necessary to rely also upon later printed sources, especially the commentaries appended to Hartmann's later editions of Oswald Croll's *Basilica chymica* and Beguin's *Tyrocinium chymicum* and Hartmann's own *Praxis chymiatrica* (all completed around the same time of the diary notations) for information helpful in revealing possible directions of laboratory work. Not everything written in the diary pertains to the work of Hartmann's students. On occasion one finds a non-laboratory reference such as an addition to chemical entries made on 27 August 1615:

"The day was Sunday. Note, on the same day, in the morning, after the address held by Dr. Schönfeld from Chapter 8 of the Epistle to the Romans, a Polish Jew named Jacob and a Jewish girl, Rahel . . . were baptized; and he received the name Christian Paul and she was called Christina Maria."[27]

Other references show Hartmann at work on what seem to be his own projects, or indicate his being away from the laboratory altogether. A note of 20 July finds laboratory operations

[27] Erlangen (n.2), p. 19.

involving the digestion and distillation of *acetum* (vinegar) and *spiritus nitri* left in the hands of a servant after Hartmann had been called away for a week to the Nassau court at Beilenstein.[28] Another entry on 7 August indicates that chemical work had ceased for three days while Hartmann visited the court at Witgenstein.[29] Later, diary notes show Hartmann traveling to the court of Nassau Catzenelenbogen, a journey that contributed to holding up work in the laboratory for almost two weeks.[30]

That Hartmann, even while serving as a courtly appointed member of the Marburg faculty, responded frequently to the invitations of princes outside Hesse was a point of concern to the Kassel prince, Moritz. In fact, suspicion that Hartmann might accept a position at the court of Anhalt-Dessau led to Moritz's personal investigation of the matter in 1618.[31] The relationship between the two was also affected by those who sought to advance their own positions at Hartmann's expense. For instance, to distract the prince from favors seemingly lavished upon the new professor of *chymiatria* one critic charged that Hartmann's loyalty was suspect and warned the Landgrave that he intended to fill his sack in Hesse and then traipse away again, leaving the country and his prince behind.[32]

Despite the digressions, the overwhelming proportion of entries in Hartmann's laboratory diary are directly concerned with daily laboratory activities. On the first day of instruction (10 July 1615) students began with the evaporation of opium. A pound of opium, cut into pieces, was placed into ten bowels (nearly enough for each student in the laboratory) and dried over the next several days. This was the first step in a careful process that would produce twenty-seven ounces of *laudanum opiatum* in six weeks. In the meantime, Hartmann instructed his students in other processes related to the laudanum preparation that produced substances having pharmaceutical uses in their own right. In order to present as coherent a picture of laboratory operations as possible, I will first sketch

[28] Erlangen (n.2), p. 6.
[29] Erlangen (n.2), p. 11.
[30] Erlangen (n.2), p. 39.
[31] Rudolf Schmitz and Adolf Winkelmann, "Johannes Hartmann (1568–1631), 'Doctor Medicus et Chymiatriae Professor Publicus,' Eine Biographisches Skizze," *Pharmazeutische Zeitung* 111(1966):1240.
[32] Murhardsche Bibliothek, Kassel: 2° MS Chem 19, vol. 1, 150r-151r.

out the calendar of procedures relating to the making of *laudanum opiatum* and then return to a discussion of accompanying processes, including directions for the making of the *aurum potabile* of Francis Anthony.

Students completed their initial drying of opium on the thirteenth of July, but further drying followed once the opium had been ground in a mortar. When the opium was determined to be uniformly dry (18 July) it was dissolved in distilled vinegar as a means of obtaining an opium extract through distillation. To make the magistery of coral, a half pound of red coral needed to be dissolved with strong distilled vinegar in a retort. Students prepared a solution of pearls in the same way. Thereafter, they filtered the two solutions separately several times, always with the addition of new vinegar, and finally (26 July) poured the two together.[33]

Another operation, completed jointly with the dissolution of corals and pearls, was the calcification of two pounds of tartar with the same measure of salt. The procedure required the mixture to be twice "detonated" in a mortar with a glowing spatula. The white salt that remained was then dissolved in water and purified by filtration.

Once the purified tartar solution had been made it could be added to the solution of coral and pearl (27 July). But at this point there was a problem. Hartmann had expected a precipitation to take place. When it did not, he surmised that not enough vinegar had been added to the solutions. Adding new vinegar, however, still did not help produce the desired precipitate and Hartmann concluded that the problem must rest with the type of container being used. Without any further commentary, the laboratory notes indicate that the desired effect was finally achieved by replacing a glass vessel with an earthen container. The superfluous phlegm formed in the process of precipitation was thereafter removed through filtering and the solution "edulcorated" (purified) seven times (29 July).[34]

For the production of laudanum, twelve ounces of *crocus martis* (oxides of iron) were put into a small linen bag and

[33] Erlangen (n.2), p. 6. Ganzenmüller, "Das chemische Laboratorium" (n.1), p. 216.

[34] Erlangen (n.2), pp. 7–8. Ganzenmüller, "Das chemische Laboratorium" (n.1), p. 216.

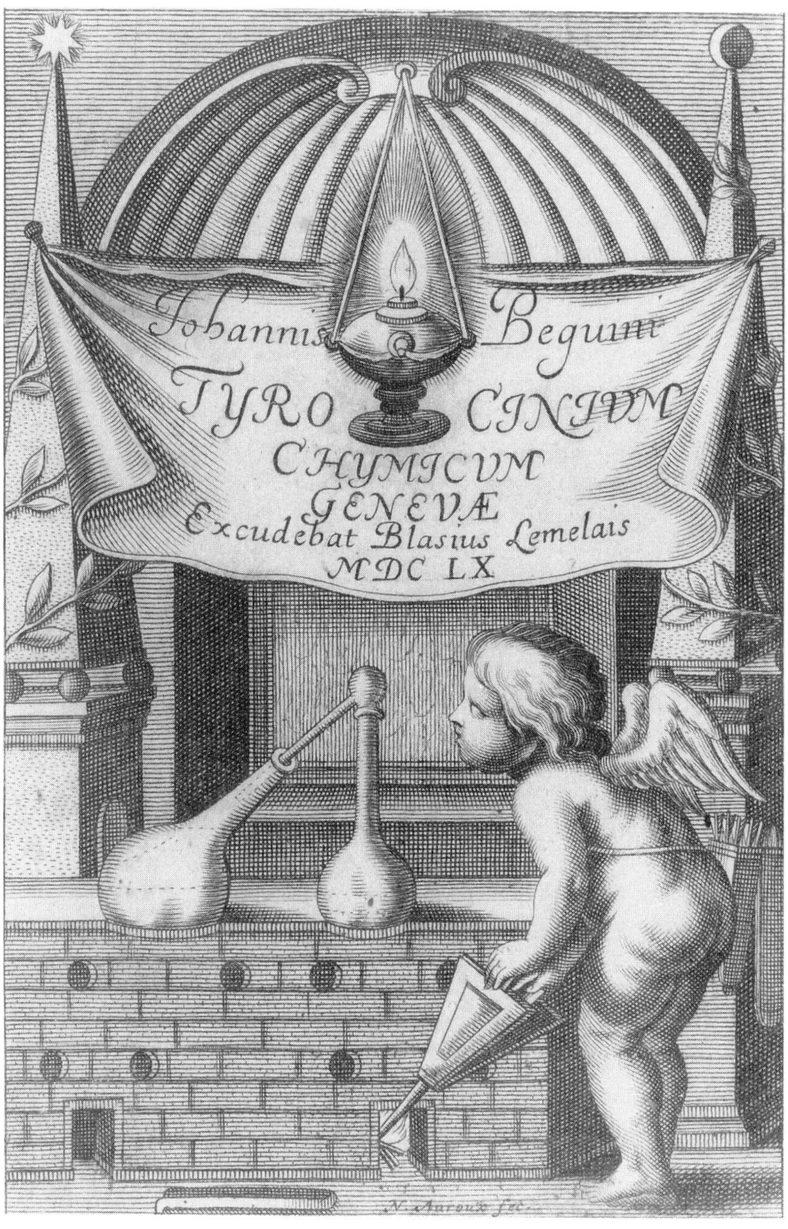

The title page of a later edition of Jean Beguin's Tyrocinium Chymicum, *edited by Hartmann under the name Christopher Glückradt.*

the bag suspended in a bladder that was then hung from an "iron cross." Hartmann and his students then carefully poured spirit of wine (alcohol) into the bladder which was then sealed. The bladder containing the bag of *crocus martis* was thereafter lowered into a warm water bath. According to Hartmann's account, the spirit of wine then rose in the bladder and penetrated the linen bag through condensation causing blood red drops to be extracted from the *crocus*. The extraction was left to continue for a week.

On the second of August students began the process of drying (evaporating) the opium extract by placing the extract in a bath of sand. At the same time, after several edulcorations, they laid out the magisteries of corals and pearls to dry in the sun. Also, the crocus extract was placed in a *Marienbad* (*balneum mariae* or water bath) in order to distill out the spirit of wine. A half pound of pearls still needed to be dissolved and the solution filtered, and the salt of tartar needed also to be dissolved, filtered, and coagulated. By mid August, students were precipitating the pearl solution with oil of tartar. Everything was ready for producing laudanum on 21 August. Hartmann showed his students how to liquify twelve ounces of opium extract in an earthen crucible over a coal fire and then how, using a spatula, to mix into the liquid extract six ounces of magistery of corals and the same amount of magistery of pearls. As a last step, students distilled three ounces of their crocus extract and added the same to the opium mixture producing a mass out of which pills could be formed.[35]

The Fullness of Instruction: The *Aurum Potabile* and the Preparation of Purgatives

It was not just the production of *laudanum opiatum* that students learned in Hartmann's course of *chymiatria*, but a variety of complementary processes as well. The magisteries of corals and pearls, essential to Hartmann's laudanum procedure, were themselves medicaments and often recommended as comfortatives. Hartmann probably recommended the procedure contained in Jean Beguin's *Tyrocinium chymicum*, a text which he himself edited under the name Chris-

[35] Erlangen (n.2), pp. 15–16. Ganzenmüller, "Das chemische Laboratorium" (n.1), p. 216.

topher Glückradt in 1618,[36] but which was not published until 1634. There, pearls or corals were to be powdered, mixed either with spirit of wine or spirit of vitriol and allowed to digest. Pouring on oil of tartar made the solution appear milky, but with the addition of water and following a second digestion a bright brown powder precipitated to the bottom of the vessel, which powder, separated from the water and gathered together, was itself the desired medicament.

Other processes also had independent pharmaceutical value. The production of spirit of vitriol (diluted sulphuric acid) and the distillation of urine from a boy who had drunk wine were begun on 11 July, the day following the first steps in the preparation of opium. Both were important procedures leading to the making of a variety of remedies and find places in the laboratory diary related to the production of *spiritus antepilepticus* (used to treat epilepsy in children) (19 July),[37] the making of an ophthalmic (2 August),[38] and, especially, in the production of the English *aurum potabile.*

Although a major focus of their laboratory contract, students had to wait until 3 August for Hartmann to fulfill his promise to instruct them in making this last medicament, the *aurum potabile.* There was no real secret about it. Already in 1610 Francis Anthony had published his own account, *Medicinae chymicae et veri potabilis auri assertio* (Cambridge, 1610) which inspired attacks by Matthew Gwynne and Thomas Rawlin in the following year.[39] By the time Hartmann began his laboratory demonstrations at Marburg, Anthony had also come to the attention of the Kassel court having entered the Landgrave Moritz's circle of alchemical correspondents in 1612.[40]

[36] A manuscript copy of Hartmann's "Annotationes in Beguinum Christophori Gluckradts," (1618) is to be found in the Deutsches Museum, Munich. The work was published as *Tyroncinium Chymicum Johannis Beguini, Regis Galliae Eleemosynarii, Antehac a Viris Clariss. Dn. Christophoro Gluckradt . . . Notis elegantibus illustratum. . .Nunc vero a Johanne-Georgio Pelshofero . . . Notis et medicamentorum formulis in unum systema redactis . . .* (Wittenberg: Georg Müller, 1634). The work appears in vol. 3 of Hartmann's *Opera Omnia* (1684).

[37] Erlangen (n.2), p. 6.

[38] Erlangen (n.2), p. 9.

[39] On Gwynne and Rawlin see Allen G. Debus, *The English Paracelsians* (New York: Franklin Watts, 1965), pp. 142–145.

[40] MBK: 2° MS Chem 19, vol. I, fol. 259r-260r.

In the notebook, the actual description of the English *aurum potabile* received far less detailed attention than the laudanum procedure.[41] Hartmann treated the panacea more fully in his *Praxis chymiatrica*, a lengthy description of pharmaceutical recipes derived in part from experiences in the Marburg laboratory, and it is to this published account that we must turn for help in trying to reconstruct what students probably encountered in Hartmann's demonstration.

The main ingredient, of course, was gold. When purified by fusion with antimony, the purified gold could next be dissolved in *aqua regis* (made from *aqua fortis* and sal ammoniac). Hartmann may then have directed adding to the solution oil of tartar until the aqua regis became clear and white. This would indicate, he notes in his *Praxis*, that all the calx (the real focus of the procedure thus far) had descended to the bottom of the vessel. After the liquid part had been poured off and the calx washed four or five times in water, Hartmann recommends that it be dried with a gentle fire. Half as much powdered sulphur was then mixed with the calx and the mixture placed in a crucible. Heating the mixture over an open fire caused the sulphur to burn leaving a very small amount of calx of gold.

Producing of the actual *aurum potabile* involved several steps of distillation. To the calx of gold first had to be added a menstruum made from spirit of wine (alcohol) and spirit of urine. The calx covered by the menstruum was then let to digest in a gentle heat until it became a bloody red. Next, Hartmann directed in the *Praxis* that as often as the menstruum became tinged it should be taken off the calx and digested in a bath so that the tinged spirit could be extracted without disturbing the feces. The salt would remain in the bottom of the vessel in the form of a red oil. In a final step, this oil was dissolved and distilled so that, Hartmann predicted, the tincture of gold will arise through the alembic leaving behind a black, dry, sooty, earth. The menstruum that came forth with the tincture of gold also produced an oil as a result of separation in a bath and that oil was the *aurum potabile*.[42]

[41] Erlangen (n.2), pp. 9–10.

[42] *Praxis chymiatrica* (n.16), in Hartmann, *Opera Omnia*, 1:pp. 12, col. 2–13, col. 1.

It is not certain how far Hartmann and his students actually progressed in the recipe. From laboratory notes it seems that only the initial step in the process was undertaken, and this only by four of Hartmann's students. The process may have suffered from a lack of materials. Still, Hartmann probably described the process in much the same fashion as he did in the *Praxis*, telling his students that the medicament worked against every disease chiefly as a diaphoretic, evacuating malignities in the body through sweat.

Several other preparations demonstrated in Hartmann's laudanum course operated primarily as diaphoretics. One was the *arcanum cardui benedicti*. Like most of the remedies taught to students in the course, this one had well known constituents, although its means of preparation varied considerably among pharmacists and iatrochemists. For example, a "water" (distillate) made from dissolved thistle (*cardus*), had by the seventeenth century become a common pharmaceutical preparation. Used as a remedy against pain in the head, as a way to break the stone, and as an antidote for the sting of the scorpion, serpent, or spider, it had gained a place in Hieronymus Braunschweig's *Book of Distillation*.[43] But the *arcanum cardui benedicti* was not a distillate, but a salt. Many fixed salts were prepared by first burning herbs to ashes. However, Beguin's *Tyrocinium chymicum* had suggested a different method whereby the salt of herbs could be extracted without calcination. In this case, *carduus benedictus* was crushed and then boiled with water until the water was half boiled away. The remainder was then pressed out of the water, strained, and boiled again until the mixture appeared as thick as honey. When set in a cool place, a crystalline salt, like gem salt (so named, says Hartmann, because the salt has a gem-like transparency), appeared at the bottom of the vessel. The remainder of the carduus juice had then to be poured off and the remaining salt washed in water of *carduus benedictus*. When dried and mixed with spirit (water) of *carduus benedictus* it became a remedy that abundantly provoked sweat.[44] To this Hartmann suggested a further step. The salt, he directed,

[43] Hieronymus Braunschweig, *Book of Distillation*, ed. Harold J. Abrahams (New York and London: Johnson Reprint Corp., 1971), pp. 108–110.

[44] *Tyrocinium chymicum* (n.36), in Hartmann, *Opera Omnia*, 3:p. 49, cols. 1–2.

should be dissolved in the spirit of the salt of niter (saltpeter) and the solution thereafter reduced to crystals.[45] In the Marburg course he also recommended adding argil (alum) to the mixture and converting the salt again into a spirit through distillation.[46]

Certainly one of the most well known ingredients among chemical physicians in making diaphoretics was *butyrum antimoni* (butter of antimony) and it is to this that Hartmann turned in his laboratory notes on 11 August.[47] There were, of course, numerous recipes for butter of antimony. Usually a solution including antimony and salt was distilled with the resulting liquid (antimony trichloride) being left thereafter to stiffen into a buttery, crystalline paste. Paracelsus described it, partly as a medicine, partly as a point of origin for other antimony preparations. By the seventeenth century, however, butter of antimony became the essential ingredient in a variety of antimony remedies, collectively referred to as *bezoardica*, that shared in common the effect of promoting sweat and urination.

The oil of butter of antimony that Hartmann showed to his students first involved fusing and then distilling crude antimony with sublimate of mercury (*mercurius sublimatus*).[48] This led to the making of cinnabar of antimony[49] from which the sulphur of antimony, described by Hartmann in his *Praxis chymiatrica* and recommended there also as a diaphoretic, could be made.[50]

Besides learning how to prepare diaphoretics, students in the summer term were also shown how to make a number of purgatives that worked as emetics as well. Nowhere in the diary does Hartmann treat the question of why purgatives operate on the body as they do. Yet in his commentary on Croll's *Basilica chymica*, he did not refrain from suggesting a reason. There Hartmann notes that the purging faculty of medicines resides not in qualities or temperaments but in the hypostatical

[45] *Praxis chymiatrica* (n.16), in Hartmann, *Opera Omnia*, 1:p. 10, col. 1.
[46] Erlangen (n.2), pp. 2–3.
[47] Erlangen (n.2), pp. 11ff.
[48] Erlangen (n.2), pp. 11–12.
[49] Erlangen (n.2), pp. 12–13; 13–15.
[50] *Praxis chymiatrica* (n.16), in *Opera Omnia*, 1:pp. 9, col. 2; 23, col. 2 - 24, col. 1. When mixed with magisteries of coral and pearls, Hartmann recommends cinnabar of antimony as useful in treating paralysis.

principles: salt, sulphur, or mercury. Such a faculty, he advises, is especially to be found in mercurial salt (*sed potius in sale mercuriali*) which explains why extracts made with the spirit of vinegar are particularly effective. As to how these medicaments actually induce catharsis, Hartmann's opinion is that they simultaneously attract the humors and excite the expulsive faculty of the body, operating by reason of a similarity of substance. In other words, either by quantity or quality they augment the humors, so that, nature being overburdened, expulsion is the result.[51]

Perhaps because he viewed the active faculty of purgation as derived in many cases from a mercurial salt, Hartmann incorporated into his summer course several demonstrations of emetics that were made from mercury. In the notebook, the precipitation of *mercurius vitae*, the sublimation of mercury, and the edulcoration of mercury were processes individually described in advance of making of *mercurius dulcis* or the *panchymagogon Quercetani*.[52] Besides finding the recipe in Quercetanus (Duchesne), the *panchymagogon* was also described by Hartmann in an addition to the original Croll text,[53] and it is from this procedure that Hartmann's demonstration in the Marburg Laboratory seems to have been derived. In the text attributed to Croll, the recipe calls for mixing sublimate mercury and crude mercury together *pars cum parte* in a stone mortar. The mixture is then to be put into a vessel which is placed in sand for eight to ten hours to sublimate. Hartmann recommends breaking the glass to separate the crude mercury that then comes forth. What remains is sublimated again three or four times so that the sublimate becomes crystalline. This mass, thereafter made into a powder, must then be washed with rose water before being used as a medicament.[54] It would, Hartmann promised, dispel all noxious humors but its oper-

[51] *Basilica chymica* (n.14), in *Opera Omnia*, 2:p. 50, col. 1.

[52] Erlangen (n.2), pp. 20–22.

[53] *Basilica chymica* (n.14), in *Opera Omnia*, 2:p. 56, cols. 1–2.

[54] Beguin, in his *Tyrocinium chymicum*, adds colcothar (the red oxide of iron usually obtained by heating ferrous sulfate) to the mixture. But Croll, and apparently also Hartmann, considered the addition unnecessary, insisting that even without any other addition crude mercury and mercury sublimate unite easily.

ation as an emetic would be increased if flowers of the butter of antimony[55] or *mercurius vitae* were added to it.[56]

Another mercury purgative, precipitate of mercury, Hartmann notes as being the same as that which many chemists call *turbith* or *turpetum*.[57] In its preparation mercury is added to rectified oil of sulphur. After the mixture has rested in sand for two days, it is distilled and the mercury precipitated into a white mass. The mass is then ground up and washed, the mercury turning into a yellow powder. When completely dried it is put into a vial with a long neck and digested for eight days. In the process the crude mercury that sticks to the upper part of the vial is to be carefully removed. What remains in the bottom is then taken out and spirit of wine is burnt over it three times. At this point the precipitate is ready for use.[58]

Mercurius dulcis and precipitate of mercury are just two of many emetics recommended by Croll and Hartmann. Although not specifically referred to in the laboratory diary, Hartmann must also have mentioned to his students another preparation in which he took a good deal of personal pride—*aqua benedicta*. This had been described by Martin Ruland as being made of crocus of metals[59] boiled in water, wine, and beer. But Hartmann had his own variation which he described in his edition of Beguin's *Tyroncinium chymicum* (chapter 12) under the title *hepar antimonii sive crocus metallorum* (liver of antimony or the crocus of metals).[60] This remedy, he claims, always works with great effect.[61]

[55] Hartmann comments in his notes to Croll that this is nothing other than the white powder that appears following precipitation of a solution made by mixing water with Butter of Antimony, *Basilica Chymica* (n.14), in *Opera Omnia*, 2:p. 57, col. 1.

[56] *Basilica Chymica* (n.14), p. 56, col. 1. A recipe for a *panchymagogon Hartmanni*, made by mixing and then sublimating *mercurius vivus* and *mercurius sublimatus*, can be found at Erlangen, Universitätsbibliothek, MS 1147.

[57] *Basilica chymica* (n.14), in *Opera Omnia*, 2:p. 50, col. 2.

[58] *Basilica chymica* (n.14), pp. 50, col. 2—51, col. 2.

[59] In his description of *aqua benedicta*, Croll notes that there is much confusion about what is called "crocus of metals." Although the basic ingredient is antimony, the method of preparation varies. In his own account, powered antimony is mixed with purified nitre that has been made liquid over a gentle fire. The mixture is then ignited by a coal or hot iron at which point a noise is given off and the crocus of metals is prepared.

[60] *Tyrocinium chymicum* (n.36), in *Opera Omnia*, 3:p. 41, col. 2.

[61] *Basilica chymica* (n.14), in *Opera Omnia*, 2:p. 48, col. 2.

Another emetic Hartmann made from either glass or crocus of antimony mixed with rose water and cinnamon powder. The recipe received specific attention as *syrupus vomitivus D. Hartmanni* (the emetic syrup of Dr. Hartmann) which, along with his *hepar antimonii* and other personal remedies, Hartmann inserted into the actual text of his annotated edition of Croll's *Basilica*.[62]

Further description of preparations shown to students in the summer quarter would try the patience of even the kindest reader. Besides the above, however, students could be found making *lapis prunellae* (potassium nitrate)[63] (26 July), preparing philosophic spirit of vitriol, and rectifying of the spirit of vitriol (1 and 2 September). Hartmann also demonstrated an *opalinum* from *mercurius vitae* (5 September) and wrapped things up in his course on 10 September after showing students the making of an *aqua cordialis*. Each of these followed well-established procedures. Yet it is also clear that on at least one occasion Hartmann used the Marburg laboratory during the summer term to investigate a less widely discussed procedure. In this instance, his interest focused on a pharmaceutical preparation made with blood.

Sympathetic Cures and Remedies Made with Blood

On 15 July Hartmann recounts in his diary receiving from the hangman the blood of a wandering monk (*circumcellio*) who had just been executed. In his notes he then describes a procedure in which the blood was poured into a retort and mixed with *spiritus salis*. Hartmann observed that the blood immediately lost its color. He then placed the mixture into a digesting oven with the aim of producing from it the *mumia aurea*,[64] that is, the vital rejuvenating force of the body that had become the focus of the sympathetic preparations of many Paracelsian physicians. Also in the *Praxis chymiatrica*, Hartmann notes that in the summer of 1615 he restored a patient

[62] *Basilica chymica* (n.14), pp. 48, col. 2—49, col. 1.

[63] Erlangen (n.2), p. 6. In his *Praxis chymiatrica* (n.16), Hartmann discusses *lapis prunellae* as a medicament treating inflammation of the kidneys. When dissolved in simple water it opens the belly and when edulcorated with sugar removes the inflammation. *Opera Omnia*, 1:p. 60, col. 2.

[64] Erlangen (n.2), p. 3. Ganzenmüller, "Das chemische Laboratorium" (n.1), p. 219.

by taking the blood of an ass and macerating into it clean linen. The effect of the medicament he explained by reference to analogy. The ass was a melancholy animal and thus signed by God as a useful pharmaceutical source in treating cases of melancholy. After macerating the linen into the blood and allowing it to dry, the cloth was steeped in water until the water was tinged with the blood's red color. This water was given to the sick man every morning for three days, which was responsible for his recovery, Hartmann claimed.[65] Later, in the winter quarter, 1615–1616, Hartmann busied himself with making yet another blood remedy, the "water of human blood."[66]

It was the Paracelsian context of Hartmann's medical and pharmaceutical thinking that made sense of signatures and analogies in nature. For Hartmann, as we have seen, a vital principle connected all the parts of the world in a single unity. Its presence is perhaps no more obvious than in another medicament made from blood, one which also was thought to operate by analogy and which became the focus of a heated controversy. The medicament was the so-called weapon salve, which operated according to Paracelsians, not by being placed on the wound itself but rather on the instrument that had caused it.

As on other occasions Hartmann responded to the criticisms of Andreas Libavius. In his commentary to Croll's *Basilica* he characterizes Libavius's arguments against the weapon salve as sophistic and his style as rough and irritating. For his own part, however, Hartmann decides to base his claims "not on sophistry . . . but on experience."[67] Experience shows, he declares, that the effects of the weapon salve are drawn from the virtues extant in all things. Although one might deplore one's ignorance in accounting for the cause of such virtues, one must, nevertheless, subscribe to them by necessity and admire their power. No one knows why wounds should be cured by this salve when the weapon, and not the wound, is treated

[65] *Praxis chymiatrica* (n.16), in *Opera Omnia*, 1:p. 15, col. 2.

[66] Reference to the water of human blood appears in Braunschweig, *Book of Distillation* (n.43), pp. 183–184. The blood of a healthy man, distilled in the middle of May, is there recommended for treating a "consumed member" of the body. When drunk, it is held to be good for consuming sicknesses of the lungs.

[67] *Basilica chymica* (n.14), in *Opera Omnia*, 2:p. 125, col. 2.

with the unguent. But as Hartmann asks, what purpose does it serve to remain blind to the manifest light of experience? After all, one knows by experience that the magnet draws iron, and yet who really understands the reason for it? The same can be said for the unguent. Indeed, Hartmann writes, we must not judge things to be among the diabolical arts simply because they run counter to our opinion.

Libavius insists on natural things. Such a view, Hartmann answers, is quite correct. But what is natural ought to extend to the sympathies of nature since a sympathy is merely a "continuation of nature" (*continuatio naturae*). Thus, while the magnet and iron are apart, nature is continued between the two so that they come together as one. No one knows the true character and source of that continuation of nature. Yet, we do not need to acquiesce in our ignorance, but we ought to try, as much as our minds are able, to understand such things. Thus the sympathy in this cure should also be explored. What has to be considered first is the subject or *materia*, which, in this case, is the blood itself. Second, one has to consider the efficient cause that is the secret *spiritus mundi* pervading all things (*quae est spiritus Mundi secretus omnia perlustrans*). The third is the instrumental cause without which a cure is not achieved.

> We say, therefore, that the basis of the martial unguent is *usnea* or coagulated corporeal animal spirit: for when a man is strangled, the vital and natural spirits are sown upwards, and these same spirits, since an exit does not lie open on account of the solid hardness of the human cranium, are closed in together through suffocation, one with the animal spirits, and are circumscribed as if by a prison, until, in the progression of time, they coalesce into one thing and burst forth at the circumference of the cranium. Thereafter, by coming upon mercury or the spirit of the world . . . *usnea*, the basis of this medicament, is made; and it contains in itself all animal, vital, and natural virtues which it communicates thereafter in the same manner to the unguent.[68]

Although the volatile spirits in the blood soon vanish into air, the spirits in the salt of the blood remain fixed in it and are not expelled. Thus, says Hartmann, when the weapon is anointed with the medicament,[69] the fixed salt of the blood draws mag-

[68] *Basilica chymica* (n.14), in *Opera Omnia*, 2:p. 126, col. 1.

[69] The salve is made as follows. The fat of a bear (or boar) is boiled in red wine and afterward poured out into cold water. Whatever settles to the bottom is thrown away. Earthworms, washed in water and wine, are next

netically and naturally (*magnetica et naturali*) the animal spirit from the salve into the sword or weapon. This spirit joins with the spirit of the world which is diffused through all things and is that which unites all things. "Hence it is that whatever . . . that coagulated spirit outside the veins senses or perceives, the same it communicates sympathetically to its own kind residing in the veins; and this does not occur except by the medium of that universal spirit renewing those things imprisoned within all bodies."[70] In this way, then, the animal spirit which is outside the man, in the blood, is communicated by the world spirit and helps, therefore, to heal the wound. How that communication actually takes place, Hartmann does not dare to explain. In such matters it is best to have an open mind. Simply because one remains ignorant of something it does not follow that "it ought forthwith be proclaimed magical. So it would certainly have to be proclaimed that the ebb and flow of the sea is magical, for, to be sure, although many causes have been advanced, still it is hitherto something unknown. The same ought to stand for infinite other things. Certainly many things lie hidden in the abyss of nature and scarcely the smallest part is fully known to us."[71]

The use of the weapon salve occasioned frequent debate, as much among hermeticists themselves as between hermetic and non-hermetic authors. In the same year that Hartmann defended chemical medicine in his inaugural as *professor publicus chymiatriae*, there appeared in print the entrance oration of another medical professor at Marburg, Rudolf Goclenius (the younger), with the title *De magnetica curatione vulneris*. Like Hartmann and other Paracelsians, Goclenius argued that the salve operated sympathetically, healing the wounded part of the body by virtue of the attractive powers extending between man and the macrocosm.

---

dried in an oven and then ground to a powder. The powder is then added to dried boar's brains, red odiferous sanders, mummy (Hartmann notes that this is the common, Egyptian sort, not *mumia patibuli* of Paracelsus), and stone hamatitis. Then one is to take *usnea* shaved off the cranium of one who has died violently (Hartmann comments that the *usnea* is better coming from someone who has been hanged). All the ingredients are beaten and mixed together with the fat thus making an unguent with which the weapon is treated. *Basilica chymica* (n.14), in *Opera Omnia*, 2:p. 124, col. 2.

[70] *Basilica chymica*(n.14), in *Opera Omnia*, 2:p. 126, col. 2.

[71] *Basilica chymica* (n.14), in *Opera Omnia*, 2:p.126, col. 2.

Soon thereafter, while students gained practical insight into the preparation of chemical medicines within the Hartmann laboratory, Goclenius's treatise, echoing also from the academic sounding board at Marburg, began to arouse distant controversy. In 1617, the work was assailed in the writings of a Jesuit pedagogue named Jean Roberti (1569–1651), leading to a controversy in which each side attacked and counterattacked over the next eight years.[72] Like Hartmann, Goclenius was particularly sensitive to the claim that the sympathetic action of the weapon salve had a diabolical origin. Sympathetic relations were, on Goclenius's view, altogether natural since all things in nature are linked by a magnetic virtue. The action of the weapon salve rested finally on the same foundations that supported the use of astrological images and talismans. Like the salve, these functioned not by the invocation of demons, but naturally as a result of astral spirits flowing into them from celestial bodies. Thus each thing in the world had its own determined counterpart in the heavens from which it received special virtues apart from those characterizing it within a particular family of objects.[73] Like all other sympathetic effects, the weapon salve depended upon astral (magnetic) virtues that supplied it with special powers that could be directed towards a particular medical purpose.

Goclenius emphasized astral connections between the wound and weapon. That, however, was not the view of either Croll or Hartmann, both of whom sought a causal link in the "continuation of nature" that arose from the blood of the victim and extended between wound and weapon. That view had much more in common with an interpretation offered by the Belgian physician J.B. van Helmont (1579–1644) in a 1621 treatise, *De magnetica vulnerum curatione*, which became van Helmont's contribution to the Goclenius-Roberti dispute.

Both Goclenius and van Helmont held to the existence of a spiritual force within matter capable of sympathetic action over distance. In van Helmont's view, however, Goclenius had erred

[72] The more important treatises in the polemic were collected together by Sylvester Rattray, *Theatrum sympatheticum auctum . . . de pulvere sympathetico . . . de unguento vero armario* (Nürnberg, 1662).

[73] D.P. Walker, *Spiritual and Demonic Magic from Ficino to Campanella* (London: Warburg Institute, University of London, 1958). Wolf-Dieter Müller-Jahncke, *Astrologisch-Magische Theorie und Praxis in der Heilkunde der frühen Neuzeit* (Stuttgart: Franz Steiner, 1985).

in arguing that the weapon salve might be applied directly to the weapon itself without the presence of the victim's blood. For the magnetic virtue to operate naturally, he insisted, objects must in some way be naturally connected. Between the sword and the wound in the body van Helmont, like Hartmann, admitted no such connection. However, when the blood of the victim remained on the sword the natural magnetic-spiritual force existing between it and the wound allowed the salve to effect a cure sympathetically, because the salve was also made, according to van Helmont, mostly also of the victim's blood.[74]

Croll's *Basilica Chymica* and the Winter Term (1615–1616)

In contrast to the summer course, the winter term (from 6 November 1615 to 10 January 1616) was concerned exclusively with the production of medicaments described by Croll in the *Basilica chymica*. Following a preliminary inscription proclaiming "Our help from Jehovah who made heaven and earth," the second part of the notebook announces itself as an *Elenchus seu diarium laborum chymicorum totius Baslicae Chymicae Oswaldi Crollii: privato collegio . . . Marburgi 1615 et 1616 dirigente Joanne Hartmanno D. Medico, chymiatriae professore publico* (*Elenchus* or diary of the chemical works of the entire *Basilica chymica* of Oswald Croll: in the private college . . . of Marburg 1615 and 1616 directed by Johann Hartmann, Medical Doctor, public professor of *chymiatria*). There follow inscriptions in Greek and Latin in which Hartmann declares to his students that "there is nothing reprehensible in the desire to know," and then pronounces the *lex huius diarii* (the law of this diary) which is that no one may keep a copy of the notebook at home and for private use for longer than one night.[75]

For the winter course Hartmann's laboratory was slightly more crowded. Sixteen students enrolled, coming, as they had also in the summer quarter, from both foreign and German-

[74] Walter Pagel, *Johann Baptista Van Helmont, Reformer of Science and Medicine* (Cambridge: Cambridge University Press, 1982), pp. 8–11. Cf. Pagel, *The Religious and Philosophical Aspects of van Helmont's Science and Medicine* (Baltimore: The Johns Hopkins Press, 1944).

[75] Erlangen (n.2), p. 29.

HERMES TRISME GISTOS ÆGYPTI
GEBER ARABS
Cherubim
Throni
Seraphim
Dominationes
Potestates
Virtutes
Principatus
Archangeli
Angeli
Pater
SANCTA TRINITAS
MESSIAS
DEVS
LVX IN ACCESSA
HOMO
Quod est Superius, est Sicut id quod est inferius
In Sole et Sale Naturæ Sunt omnia.
D·O·M·A·
MORIENES ROMANVS
ROG. BACCHON ANGLUS
OSUALDI CROLLII VETERANI HASSI
BASILICA CHYMICA
CONTINENS,
Philosophicam propriâ laborum experientiâ confirmatam descriptionem et usum Remediorum Chymicorum Selectissimorum é Lumine GRATIÆ et NATURÆ DESUMPTORUM.
In fine libri additus est Autoris ejusdem Tractatus Nouus DE SIGNATURIS Rerum Internis.
Occultum fiat manifestum, et viceuersa
Per elementorum conuersionem Ternarius purificatus fiat MONAS
R. LULLIUS HISPANUS
TH. PARACELSVS GERMANUS.
LUMINIS NATURÆ BONUM FINITUM
ORA ET LABORA REPUTANS OMNIA VANA PRETER AMARE DEUM ET ILLI SOLI SERVIRE.
CABALA THEOLOGICA MAGIA ASTRONOMICA HALCHYMIA MEDICA
Ignis
ANIMA
Animalia
Terra
Mineralia
Vegetabilia
CORPUS
SPIRITUS
Aqua
Aer
Cum Igne tandem in gratiam redit Aqua.
Separate et ad maturitatem perducite.

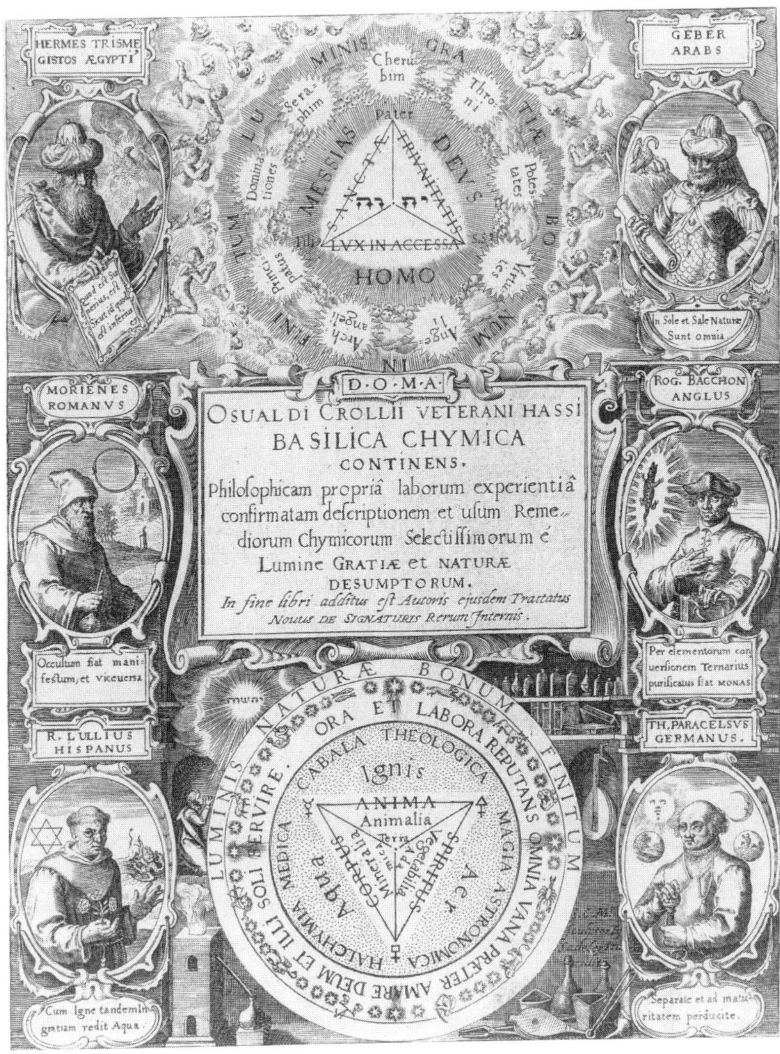

Title page of Croll's Basilica chymica *(1609).*

speaking lands.[76] Ten students returned from the summer course. Among the rest there were present a medical doctor, Johann Jacobus, from Metz and an English nobleman, Anthony Staffort. To these Hartmann explained that the work in the laboratory would not be taken up in the same order as in Croll's text (which listed medicaments according to *vomitiva*, *cathartica*, *diuretica*, *diaphoretica*, etc.). The reason was that certain *menstrua* (dissolving agents) that were necessary for the demonstration of operations did not appear until later in Croll's book. These, however, needed to be prepared first so that as many preparations as possible could be undertaken in the time allowed.[77]

Whatever the order, the winter course was to be mostly concerned with the making of purgatives. Hartmann's own medical practice was in large part based on the use of purging remedies and in the preface to his *Praxis chymiatrica* he acknowledged that the making of such medicaments was as important to the skilled physician as diagnostic understanding. Two things, he insisted, were necessary for physicians to advance in the practice of *chymiatria*. The first was to understand the nature of disease, which meant deriving medical knowledge *ex pathologia*. The second was to understand treatment which he described as knowledge *ex therapeusi*. To treat illness the physician must comprehend pharmacy so that, Hartmann continues, he may always have at hand a good choice of remedies. There are, of course, numerous preparations, but of them all *chymica* are the most beneficial. The reason is that in the practice of medicine that which is most often sought is

[76] Erlangen (n.2), p. 31. These are Johann Jacobus from Metz D. Med., Antonius Staffort from England (nobilis), M. Hildebrandus Küen, M. Petrus Titius from Striegau in Schlesien, Nicolaus Fossius and Johannes Rhodius (both from Denmark), Paul-Pauli Cleophe from Prussia, Michael Volchmann Aurimontanus (i.e. from Goldberg) in Silesia, Daniel Becker from Danzig, Johann Stellius from Marienburg in Silesia, Simon Batkovius from Poland, Andreas Lipius from Berlin in the Mark, M. Johann Salvius Suecus, Johannes Ebelingk from Hamburg, Paulus Nuquerius from Poland, Franciscus Joelius from Sunda-Pomeranus.

[77] Erlangen (n.2), p. 31. For a discussion of the recipes of Croll's *Basilica chymica* see Monika Klutz, *Die Rezepte in Oswald Crolls Basilica chymica (1609) und ihre Beziehungen zu Paracelsus*, Veröffentlichungen aus dem Pharmaziegeschichtlichen Seminar der Technischen Universität Braunschweig, no. 14 (Braunschweig: Technische Universität, Pharmaziegeschichtliches Seminar, 1974).

evacuation. Since nature is accustomed to expel disease from the body through four avenues (i.e., through the upper and lower parts, through urine, and through the skin) the physician likewise must create emetics, purges, diuretics, and diaphoretics either from vegetables or minerals according to differences of subject and illness. Hartmann also adds that, whether on account of human weakness or the intensity of pain, comfortatives and anodynes must sometimes also be used in advance of particular cures.[78]

The preparation of *chymica* in the winter term began with the calcination of vitriol and the production of oil of vitriol. Students were also early involved with the distillation of urine (8 Nov.), the calcination of copper (13 and 14 Nov.), the extraction of copper vitriol from the calx of copper, and its filtration.[79]

In making copper vitriol Croll instructed that the whole operation consisted in calcining copper (sometimes also iron) with sulphur. The procedure was to place pieces of copper (and iron) on top of one another with powdered sulphur in between. The layers were placed in a pot (*in tigillo lutato*), the pot placed over a fire, and the heat of the fire gradually increased. After about an hour the blackened matter in the pot was removed, ground, sifted, and placed into an open earthen vessel. To every pound of calx Croll recommended adding three lots of sulphur so that, with more heating, the copper would become soft like paste. Such details are not given in Hartmann's diary, but if students followed Croll's procedure they would have allowed the mixture then to cool before repeating several more times the process of grinding, heating, and adding more sulphur. The final calx would have been ground very fine and then dissolved in hot water. When the water had turned blue they would have evaporated it until what remained became crusted and, when cooled, crystallized. These feces they would have once again calcined with sulphur, collecting the vitriol by allowing water to leach through the calx. The final product was an oil of vitriol having numerous medicinal uses. It helped, said Croll, in cases of the stone or gravel, in fevers of the stomach, in all diseases of the head, in jaundices, and in cases of the plague.[80]

[78] *Praxis chymiatrica* (n.16), in *Opera Omnia*, 1:p. 3.
[79] Erlangen (n.2), pp. 33–35.
[80] *Basilica chymica*(n.14), in *Opera Omnia*, 2:pp. 100, col. 1—101, col. 2.

Hartmann, in notes appended to Croll's text, described another way of preparing vitriol in which what he called *vitriolum hermaphroditicum* (vitriol of iron) was made following a recipe of Basilius Valentinus. This procedure was probably also explained to students in the Marburg laboratory since reference to it appears as well in the *Praxis chymiatrica* as the "greatest secret in all uterine affects, especially in the inordinate flux of the menses," and since Hartmann took pride in having brought about the cure of the Hessian Landgravine by its use.[81] Having made the oil of vitriol in the manner described by Croll, Hartmann poured the oil, mixed with three times as much rain water, onto iron filings. After filtering the solution, there remained a green liquor that produced a green vitriol when evaporated and left to cool.[82]

In everything having to do with administering oil of vitriol, both Croll and Hartmann urged extreme caution. Croll, in fact, makes reference to a certain wicked chemist who brought about the death of a good man by using too much oil of vitriol. Hartmann accuses Thomas Erastus, a Paracelsian opponent and critic of the writings of Petrus Severinus, of killing a doctor and a councilor to the prince of the Palatinate.[83] Paracelsians and Galenists were fond of trading barbs about the carnage caused by each other's medical procedures. Indeed, Hartmann was himself not immune to such attacks. During the same time that he demonstrated diaphoretics and emetics to students, the death of one of his patients led to a lawsuit in which Hartmann was accused of overzealous use of purgatives. The result of the affair is not known. However, the proceedings seem to have so soured Hartmann against his colleagues at Marburg that in 1618 the rector of the university joined university deans and fellow professors in writing to the Landgrave complaining that Hartmann had conducted himself disrespectfully toward almost everyone. The question put to Moritz was whether, given such behavior, it was to the advantage of the university to allow him to remain on the faculty.[84]

Within the arsenal of purgatives available to chemical physicians, diuretics were among the most frequently employed.

[81] *Praxis chymiatrica*(n.16), in *Opera Omnia*, 1:p. 67, col. 2.
[82] *Basilica chymica* (n.14), in *Opera Omnia*, 2:p.102, col. 1.
[83] *Basilica chymica* (n.14), in *Opera Omnia*, 2:p. 102, col. 1.
[84] Schmitz-Winkelmann, "Johannes Hartmann (1568–1631)" (n.31), pp. 1238–1240.

One of the most common was called the "spirit of salt" and it is with its preparation that students in the laboratory were occupied on 16 Nov.[85] Croll's *Basilica chymica* provided the basis for the procedure. Rain water mixed with fresh argil or with a liquor made from *terra sigillata* was to be added to sea salt and the solution distilled.[86] Hartmann commented, however, that the spirit of salt would be better made if, with sea salt, Spanish, or French salt mixed with crude *terra sigillata*, in three or fourfold proportions, was distilled over a strong, open fire. At the same time he recommended another, purer spirit of salt, the *spiritus salis compositus*, that was compounded of nitre and common salt.[87]

On 17 November, following the rectification of oil of vitriol, students were shown how to purify the oil of tartar in preparation for the making of vitriol of tartar (*tartarus vitriolatus*), which was held to be a universal digestive.[88] Croll's instructions required that salt of tartar be mixed with water of agrimony and this, thereafter, be dissolved into an oil (oil of vitriol).[89] The oil of vitriol was to be then mixed, drop by drop, with oil of tartar and the coagulate dried over a gentle heat to the consistency of a salt. Hartmann's recipe, added to Croll's own,[90] involved first extracting the salt of tartar by distilling calcined tartar mixed in rain water. To the extract he added spirit of vitriol which, after evaporation, left a mass like little stones in the bottom of the vessel, which was the vitriolate tartar.

Demonstrations concerning *tartarus vitriolatus* began on 20 November. On the same day students learned how to make *aqua fortis* for the purpose of sublimating mercury. Those students who had also been enrolled in the summer term would have already experienced the making of sublimate mercury and so Hartmann's sudden withdrawal from the laboratory for the period of almost two weeks, during which time he paid a medical visit to one of the Nassau courts, was possibly less disappointing than for others expecting to make regular progress in chemical preparations. Hartmann, however, did not

[85] Erlangen (n.2), p. 36.
[86] *Basilica chymica* (n.14), in *Opera Omnia*, 2:pp. 67, col. 2—68, col. 2.
[87] *Basilica chymica* (n.14), in *Opera Omnia*, 2:pp. 68, col. 2-2-69, col. 1.
[88] Erlangen (n.2), pp. 36–37.
[89] *Basilica chymica* (n.14), in *Opera Omnia*, 2:p. 45, col. 1.
[90] *Basilica chymica* (n.14), in *Opera Omnia*, 2:pp. 45, col. 2 -46, col. 2.

return until 8 December at which time the focus of instruction changed to the making of *galbani balsamus*. This was a medicament especially praised in the treatment of paralysis. Galbanum was to be mixed with spirit of turpentine and digested for eight days. Thereafter an extract could be gathered by distillation. Perhaps because the odor of galbanum was unpleasant, Hartmann advised rectifying the dried extract with nutmeg and cassia.[91]

As in the first term, Hartmann also emphasized the making of diaphoretics in the winter course. Once again he instructed students how to make *mercurius dulcis* (*panchymagogum Quercetani*) beginning his description in earnest on 12 Dec. Thereafter, he once more took up the antimony remedies—especially butter of antimony and *cinnabaris antimonii*.[92] Students were involved with these and other diaphoretic medicaments throughout the rest of December and into January 1616. Along the way they also prepared red flowers of antimony (*flores antimonii rubei*), according to Croll, by sublimating the powder of antimony mixed with sand.[93] They also made antimony's white flowers, to produce from them an oil or "strong water" (30 Dec.).

The new year found students making *bezoardicum simplex*, the especially popular antimony diaphoreticum of Croll.[94] Croll described its preparation as beginning with grinding together sublimate of mercury with vitriol, salt, and antimony. Following Croll's recipe, once distilled and rectified the resulting liquor would need to be wholly dissolved in *aqua regis*. Next, gold, also dissolved in *aqua regis* was poured into the original mixture and the combined solution placed in a cucurbit. Croll recommended heating it with a gentle fire to abstract a phlegm. From the residue that remained the medicament was made.[95]

Hartmann, for his part, did not hold the addition of gold to be necessary. He reasoned that in the process gold was reduced to its pristine body and therefore could not be an active agent.

[91] Erlangen (n.2), pp. 40–41. *Praxis chymiatrica* (n.16) in *Opera Omnia*, 1:pp. 23, col. 2—24, col. 1.

[92] Erlangen (n.2), pp. 42ff.

[93] Erlangen (n.2), p. 45. *Basilica chymica* (n.14), in *Opera Omnia*, 2:pp. 58, col. 2—59. col. 1.

[94] Erlangen (n.2), pp. 57–60.

[95] *Basilica chymica* (n.14), in *Opera Omnia*, 2:p. 70, cols. 1–2.

Thus, contrary to Croll's contention, it could never render the powder of antimony more virtuous. On the other hand, Hartmann did recommend a "solar bezoar," described as antimony mixed with gold after the gold had been reduced to a spiritual substance through repeated dissolutions and distillations in a hermetically closed retort.[96]

Both Hartmann and Croll held mineral bezoar or diaphoretic antimony to be one of the principal *arcana* in the formularies of chemical physicians. Its ability to induce sweat and urine without purging was well known. Other Paracelsian physicians including Joseph Duchesne had experimented with its preparation. However, Hartmann felt that no one had searched out the remedy as much as himself after being inspired by reading Basilius Valentinus's treatment of antimony in the *Philosophical Keys*. "For from salt-peter, [which is] the serpent of rocks (*der Steinschlangen*), with common salt, [known as] the best spice (*das beste Gewürtz*), he [Basilius] makes a water; by whose benefit, either alone, or with *aqua regis*, that exceedingly corrosive butter (of antimony) is plainly mortified, and is converted into a bezoardic powder."[97]

Discussing diaphoretic antimony provided Hartmann with yet another chance to strike out at his primary adversary, Andreas Libavius. Hartmann remarks that in explicating the mineral bezoar, Libavius had made it his business to carp rather than to inquire (*id quod magis carpendi quam inquirendi studio facit*). In particular Hartmann points to Libavius's treatment of bezoar in the second volume of his *Chemical Secrets* and in the same volume of his *Apocalypseos Hermeticae*. In these places, Hartmann writes, "this is certain:

> that Libavius, as in other things, so also in the preparation of this bezoardic, judges like Argos; that is [he is] clear sighted when abroad; but at home, he is like Tiresias. Truly he has never joined his talkative tongue with chemical experience, or, if he has done so, it has not been as a good artificer. Therefore I do not admire the shameless writing of the man and perhaps it may be publicly shown whether he shall have been so much in the laboratory as he professes."[98]

Publicly showing Libavius to be mistaken in chemical *praxis* was, as discussed above, part of the hidden agenda of Hart-

[96] *Basilica chymica* (n.14), in *Opera Omnia*, 2:p. 71, col. 2.
[97] *Basilica chymica* (n.14), in *Opera Omnia*, 2:p. 71, col. 1.
[98] *Basilica chymica* (n.14), in *Opera Omnia*, 2:p. 71, col. 1.

mann's course in *chymiatria* at Marburg. Thus, when it came to the correct preparation of diaphoretics, especially to the making of *antimonium diaphoreticum*, it is quite likely that his students not only learned what their teacher felt to be correct procedure, but also where he considered Libavius's recommendations to be in error.

Another diaphoretic found mentioned both in the summer and winter terms was *spiritus vitrioloi philosophicus*,[99] which was also sometimes used as an odorific. Pouring cold water onto butter of antimony allowed the water to "imbibe" the corrosive force of antimony's salts. When delivered of its "phlegm" by evaporation it rendered a spirit of vitriol that Hartmann called philosophic vitriol. Hartmann writes in his notes to Croll's *Basilica chymica* that it mitigates the fevers of *lues venera*, and is wonderfully useful in treating epilepsy and all affects of the head. Its preparation, however, is known to very few. It had an additional property that was attractive to the Marburg company. It could also extract the tinctures of minerals and be used to dissolve corals and pearls.[100]

Just such a dissolving agent was needed in the making of *arcanum perlarum* (15 Dec.).[101] This was an extraction from powdered pearls mixed with spirit of *lignum guaiacum*, which was described by Croll as a comfortative.[102] Of a very different nature was a medicament referred to as the *arcanum corallinum* of Paracelsus which was administered usually as a cathartic.[103] Although seemingly made from coral or coralline (*corallina*), the *arcanum corallinum* was described by Croll as the red sublimate of mercury made by sublimating mercury with saltpeter.[104] It was especially useful, advised Croll, in treating dropsy, the French sickness, and gout.

[99] Erlangen (n.2), pp. 22–23.
[100] *Basilica chymica* (n.14), in *Opera Omnia*, 2:pp. 57, col. 2; 89, col. 2.
[101] Erlangen (n.2), pp. 44–45.
[102] *Basilica chymica* (n.14), in *Opera Omnia*, 2:p. 78, col. 1.
[103] Erlangen (n.2), pp. 54ff.
[104] The origin of the recipe was disputed among chemists and chemical physicians. Libavius denied that Paracelsus was the author, thinking that its origin could be traced either to Croll or to Johann Heuser. Hartmann also viewed Heuser as connected to the process, believing that in his works the original recipe of Paracelsus had lain hidden for a long time before finally coming to light. *Basilica chymica* (n.14), in *Opera Omnia*, 2:p. 54, col. 2.

Although chemical remedies predominated in the winter quarter, the preparation of vegetable based medicaments were also included among laboratory demonstrations. Shortly before Christmas 1615, students began preparing *balsamus aloetici* which was made by distilling ground aloe mixed with *aqua betonicae*.[105] Following a one-day Christmas vacation students returned to this recipe and attended at the same time to others. In particular they made a *lixivium* of the salt of absinth (wormwood),[106] prepared *aqua cinnai*,[107] oil of sulphur, and the white flowers of antimony, sublimated *mercurius dulcis*, and made butter of antimony. Finally, on 29 December Hartmann turned the attention of his students to the making of a special remedy, the *panchymagogum vegetabilis*.[108]

This last medicament, invented supposedly by Isaac Holland and repeated by Beguin, found a place also in Hartmann's *Praxis chymiatrica*. There it is described as made from the pulp of coloquintida (*cucumus colocynthis*), leaves of sena orient, rhubarb, wallwort seeds, root of black hellebore, agaric, cinnamon, and cloves. These, he advises, should be steeped in spirit of wine followed by digestion over sixteen days so that the spirit of wine becomes well tinged. Having repeated this procedure until no more tincture is given off, one is then ready to pour spirit of wine with a few drops of oil of tartar and oil of sulphur over elaterium (from the juice of wild cucumbers) and the juice of aloes. The mixture must then be set in a warm place in a closed vessel for a few days and filtered. The second extract is then to be added to the first. Finally, Hartmann instructs that scammony should be mixed with spirit of vitriol and oil of anise seeds and worked into pitch-like mass. The mass must be evaporated with rose of majora water until dry and then added to the extracts already made before the combined extracts are formed into pills. Taken in doses of from eight grains to one

[105] Beton water (water of betony) finds a place, among others, in Braunschweig, *Book of Distillation* (n.43), pp. 93–95, where it is held to be good against pain in the head, stone in the bladder, and a large number of other ailments.

[106] Erlangen (n.2), pp. 47f.

[107] Laboratory notes call for mixing *aqua cinnai* with Pucinum wine and leaving the mixture to digest overnight in a cucurbit. Thereafter it was to be distilled through an alembic. Erlangen (n.2), p. 48.

[108] Erlangen (n.2), pp. 51–52; 58.

scruple the medicine, says Hartmann, is a gentle purging extract.[109]

Hartmann's diary account of making the medicament differs slightly from this one. In adding notes to Croll's *Basilica chymica*, he records the very recipe worked out in December 1615 in the Marburg laboratory. There, Hartmann adds to the mixture the piths of carthamus seeds, hermodactyls, aromatic caryophyllata, diamber, the rinds of citron, balsam of aloe, and (turning away from purely vegetable components) the magisteries of pearls and corals.[110]

The last weeks of the winter term were especially busy. Students, knowing the end of term was close at hand, hurried to prepare the flowers of antimony. At the same time, they distilled, corrected, and edulcorated the butter of antimony, extracted *balsam aloetici*, made *aqua fortis* and *arcanum corallinum*, and also extracted *panchymagogon vegetabilis*. To end the course Hartmann demonstrated the spirit of treacle water (*aqua theriacalis*) which he described as a Paracelsian diaphoretic of much use in treating victims of the plague.[111]

[109] The recipe follows generally that which is recorded by Beguin in his *Tyroncinium chymicum* (n.36), chapter 9, "extracts." *Praxis chymiatrica* (n.16), in *Opera Omnia*, 1:pp. 6, col. 2—7, col. 2.

[110] *Basilica chymica* (n.14), in *Opera Omnia*, 2:pp. 62, col. 2—63, col. 1.

[111] Erlangen (n.2), pp. 64–65. Also, *Basilica chymica* (n.14), in *Opera Omnia*, 2:p. 106, cols. 1–2. Here Hartmann notes, in commenting upon Croll's discussion of pestilentials, that no specific remedy can expel the plague. Whatever the physician might try, therefore, if God does not will it, shall be in vain. Nevertheless, Hartmann also notes his own use of a certain *aqua pestilentialis* during a severe outbreak in Hesse in 1611. It seemed to him that tiny bits of the disease could be seen flying in the air [*habenas in aere volantes*] (p. 104, col. 2). That infection resulted from tiny pieces of corrupt matter was a notion popular in the Renaissance. See Vivian Nutton, "The Seeds of Disease: An Explanation of Contagion and Infection from the Greeks to the Renaissance," *Medical History* 27(1983):1–34. Treacle water is also discussed in Hartmann's *Praxis chymiatrica* (n.16), *Opera Omnia*, 1:pp. 10, col. 2—11, col. 1.

Conclusion

It is worth pointing out once again that none of Hartmann's laboratory procedures appeared in print during his lifetime. The lack of publication disturbed one of his closest friends, Wilhelm Dilich, who explained that Hartmann had intentionally held back his work from print so as to distance his procedures from the uninformed, vulgar sort of alchemical-medical literature that he saw as having become widespread.[112] Dilich's explanation was probably less correct than another, however, namely that Hartmann viewed his procedures as somehow privileged information and made every attempt to keep them as such. That laboratory procedure should be a form of privileged knowing was a view of pharmaceutical knowledge connected, on the one hand, to a secretive tradition of alchemical discussion, but included social and economic motives as well. For Hartmann, the latter were far more important. He viewed the communication of laboratory procedures as *privatim dictans* (private conversation), which protected his own financial well being as well as his special stature with his ultimate patron, the Hessian prince, Moritz. The interesting thing is that as privileged as chemical-medical knowledge was held to be, it was also readily provided once the threshold of Hartmann's laboratory had been crossed. There attention to Hartmann's Severinian-based Paracelsian philosophy was of less importance to students than minding the heat of the fire and participating in the myriad tasks necessary in preparing medicines chosen for demonstration. Students learned to value their teacher's practical skills. They may also have come to respect his philosophy, especially since Hartmann's laboratory

[112] Rudolf Schmitz, *Die Naturwissenschaften an der Philipps-Universität Marburg* (Marburg: N. G. Elwert), p. 196.

successes were sometimes displayed together with reference to the supposed inabilities of his primary philosophical antagonist, Andreas Libavius.

Important as well from the point of view of the agreed upon secrecy of laboratory work is the fact that, besides teaching *chymiatria* within the medical faculty, Hartmann also continued a private medical practice. The remedies which he provided, if considered as something akin to professional secrets, added to the desirability of his consultation. As several references in the laboratory diary indicate, Hartmann eagerly accommodated those seeking his medical assistance, especially when the desire for it came from court.

Hartmann knew that good things could come from courtly patronage. The discipline of *chymiatria*, whatever its value to the Marburg medical curriculum, had arisen primarily due to the support of the Kassel court. There the Hessian prince, Moritz, doled out social privileges and financial rewards to those proclaiming his own mystical-alchemical court philosophy. Hartmann, like many others in Kassel and Marburg, was close at hand when Moritz required alchemical-medical advice. In 1621 his service to Moritz became closer still when he accepted a courtly invitation to become the prince's personal physician. For all practical purposes, teaching *chymiatria* as a specific laboratory course came to an end at Marburg with Hartmann's departure, although pharmacy, including instruction in the making of chemical medicaments, continued to find a place in the medical curriculum owing to the continued presence there of one of Hartmann's students, Johann Phillipp Molther.

The reasons for Hartmann's withdrawal from the university are not known. Perhaps he had simply grown weary of the routine of lecture and laboratory demonstration. Or perhaps by 1621 personal animosities with fellow professors had made continuation at the university unbearable. Hartmann was at times difficult to get along with. His independent character seemed arrogant to some. But if Moritz insisted that his behavior be tolerated at the university, he would have none of it at the Kassel court. Indeed, Hartmann found himself in hot water soon after his arrival there. Rumors about his intellectual and personal loyalties rather quickly made their way to the ear of the Landgrave. Moritz, who valued his physician's laboratory skills for alchemical reasons, was told that Hartmann considered alchemical procedures relating to transmutation to be a waste of time. He also heard that Hartmann had held clandestine conversations in which he supposedly had made utterances against the prince.[113] Where all else might be accepted, suspicion that Hartmann no longer supported the intellectual values of his prince's court was not. Hartmann found himself faced with the loss of his court position and its accompanying stipend. He explained that he had not actually doubted the attainability of transmutation itself, but had only questioned the ability of a certain procedure being tried in one of the court laboratories to achieve it. Neither had he ever expressed anything but praise and affection for his patron.[114] Moritz, although angered, was satisfied with the explanation; and Hartmann knew that for his part, his value at court was measured as much by alchemical as by medical expertise. Letters that survive in Kassel from this period reveal the double expectation of medical and alchemical service. He reports on the health and treatment of the princely family and offers a detailed account of an outbreak of dysentery within the city of Kassel. But Hartmann also adds references to alchemical procedures. His letters now bear the seal of the *Monas*, the symbol of unity connected to a Renaissance Platonic and alchemical view of nature. In them a main concern is to answer questions put to him by the prince concerning alchemical-pharmaceutical *particularia*. He discusses English potable gold, the processes of Duchesne, the *arcanum vitriolis*, the preparation of philosophical mercury, as well as the "best tincture of gold" and its multiplication.[115]

Even at court, Hartmann's role was partially pedagogical. In contrast to his position at Marburg, however, he did not have to defend his Paracelsian medical philosophy. That Hartmann could function as well within alchemical circles at court as within the medical faculty at Marburg gives, I think, added weight to what many have suspected before, namely, that at least part of the way from alchemy to chemistry leads through a particular chapter in the history of pharmacy. Alchemy itself was, in many ways, a pharmaceutical enterprise. But *chymiatria*, however short its career as a discipline at Marburg,

[113] Murhardsche Bibliothek, Kassel: 2° MS Chem 19, 3: 109r–111r.
[114] Murhardsche Bibliothek, Kassel: 2° MS Chem 19, 3: pp. 109r–v.
[115] Murhardsche Bibliothek, Kassel: 2° MS Chem 19, 5: 12r–14r.

showed that an alchemically based system of thought geared to a highly mystical philosophy of nature could claim an academic place. It was, however, the laboratory that provided that place, and although Hartmann may have wished that students would equate practical-laboratory success with the soundness of his own theoretical views, doing so was not a requirement for the purpose of learning laboratory procedures. Those instructed by Hartmann at Marburg did not have to wait for Platonic enlightenment to learn *chymiatria*, even though its epistemological foundations were firmly rooted in the philosophy of personal inspiration. Emphasizing the operational separability of Paracelsian theory and practice in this way is important. It allows us still to find a place for a Paracelsian didactic along side the well documented tradition of humanist chemical discourse in the development of chemistry in the seventeenth century. *Chymiatria* brought together traditions both ancient and modern, theoretical and practical. At Marburg it received its social legitimation from both court and university. Most important, however, in Hartmann's *laboratorium publicum chymico-medicum*, it evolved into an institutionalized, empirically based approach to chemical and pharmaceutical learning. We have also seen that Hartmann's course in *chymiatria* contained a hidden agenda. Students allowed into the laboratory entered not just a didactic space, but a polemical one as well. Libavius may have considered that, on epistemological grounds, Hartmann's presence in the Marburg faculty amounted to a corruption of one of the principal institutions of learning. Hartmann knew, however, that controlling the new discipline had both didactic and apologetic value. The response to Libavius included making official space for the medical philosophy Libavius attacked and demonstrating in that space—the *laboratorium*—the practical effectiveness of medicines derived from the medical thinking he condemned. Hartmann knew that the position and the space assigned to him within the Marburg academy raised his social status and made respectable the ideas that he represented. That they also provided him with a polemical advantage in a war not just of words is important to bear in mind when evaluating the fullness of strategies in the chemical-pharmaceutical debates of the early seventeenth century.